AF560767

Facelift

Thomas Procedures in Facial Plastic Surgery

Facelift

Thomas Procedures in Facial Plastic Surgery

J. Regan Thomas MD
Professor and Head
Department of Otolaryngology—Head and Neck Surgery
University of Illinois at Chicago
Chicago, Illinois, USA

Clinton D. Humphrey MD
Assistant Professor
Division of Facial Plastic and Reconstructive Surgery
Department of Otolaryngology—Head and Neck Surgery
The University of Kansas Medical Center
Kansas City, Kansas, USA

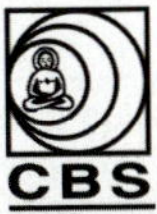

CBS Publishers & Distributors Pvt Ltd

New Delhi • Bengaluru • Pune • Kochi • Chennai
Mumbai • Kolkata • Hyderabad • Patna • Manipal

People's Medical Publishing House—USA, Shelton, Connecticut

People's Medical Publishing House-USA
2 Enterprise Drive, Suite 509
Shelton, CT 06484
Tel: 203-402-0646
Fax: 203-402-0854
E-mail: info@pmph-usa.com

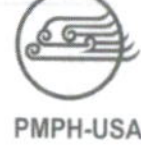

11 12 13 14/PMPH/9 8 7 6 5 4 3 2 1
ISBN-13: 978-1-60795-154-4
ISBN-10: 1-60795-154-1

This Edition has been published by special arrangement with PMPH-USA, Ltd
CBS ISBN: 978-81-239-2248-5

Special Indian Edition: 2013

Published by Satish Kumar Jain for
CBS Publishers & Distributors Pvt Ltd
4819/XI Prahlad Street, 24 Ansari Road, Daryaganj, New Delhi 110 002, India.
Ph: 23289259, 23266861, 23266867 Fax: 011-23243014 Website: www.cbspd.com
e-mail: delhi@cbspd.com; cbspubs@airtelmail.in

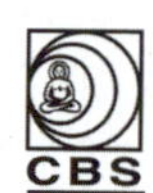

Corporate Office: 204 FIE, Industrial Area, Patparganj, Delhi 110 092
Ph: 4934 4934 Fax: 4934 4935 e-mail: publishing@cbspd.com; publicity@cbspd.com

Branches

- **Bengaluru:** Seema House 2975, 17th Cross, K.R. Road, Banasankari 2nd Stage, Bengaluru 560 070, Karnataka
  Ph: +91-80-26771678/79 Fax: +91-80-26771680 e-mail: bangalore@cbspd.com
- **Pune:** Bhuruk Prestige, Sr. No. 52/12/2+1+3/2 Narhe, Haveli (Near Katraj-Dehu Road Bypass), Pune 411 041, Maharashtra
  Ph: +91-20-64704058, 64704059, 32342277 Fax: +91-20-24300160 e-mail: pune@cbspd.com
- **Kochi:** 36/14 Kalluvilakam, Lissie Hospital Road, Kochi 682 018, Kerala
  Ph: +91-484-4059061-65 Fax: +91-484-4059065 e-mail: cochin@cbspd.com
- **Chennai:** 20, West Park Road, Shenoy Nagar, Chennai 600 030, Tamil Nadu
  Ph: +91-44-26260666, 26208620 Fax: +91-44-45530020 e-mail: chennai@cbspd.com

Representatives

- **Mumbai** 0-9833017933
- **Kolkata** 0-9831437309
- **Hyderabad** 0-9885175004
- **Patna** 0-9334159340
- **Manipal** 0-9742022075

Printed at R P Printers, Noida

To my residents and fellows who challenge my concepts and inspire me to grow and improve;

To Ryan, Aaron, and Evan Thomas, who expand my world and inspire me to enjoy it beyond what I ever imagined possible.

To M. Eugene Tardy, who demonstrates a high threshold of excellence and inspires me through example as to what a physician should be.

To Jim Thomas, who provides throughout my life examples of integrity, leadership, responsibility, humor, and continues to inspire me as my hero.

Acknowledgments

Few, if any, publications of significance are the product of single individuals. This book as a component volume of the Procedures in Facial Plastic Surgery series is no exception and benefits from the talents of numerous individuals. My gratitude is acknowledged here in this form, and I hope they indeed recognize my genuine appreciation.

Denise McManaman, devoted and dedicated assistant who demonstrated great patience with the manuscript while demonstrating great skill at keeping me organized and properly directed.

Chet Childs and Eric Johnson, for their photographic and videographic skills and assistance.

Natalie Steele Higgins, MD, for her assistance as a Fellow with anatomic demonstrations and assistance with development of the book.

Rhonda Churchill Thomas, who has provided a lifetime of devotion, encouragement, inspiration, and patience. She continues to set the standard for beauty.

Preface

Individuals interested in altering their facial appearance possess a unique set of motivating factors distinct from patients requiring surgery related to illness and abnormal pathology. Treatments for elective aesthetic goals require specific analysis and evaluation with a high standard maintained to avoid complication or untoward treatment results. This patient group is healthy psychologically as well as socially motivated to rejuvenate the results of the aging process. They are typically less prepared to accept risk or complication than the individual requiring nonelective surgery. Techniques to help serve their desire to improve and rejuvenate their appearance must minimize morbidity and possible unfavorable postoperative sequelae.

This text describes a technique that strives to combine surgical steps that minimize complications with the opportunity for excellent results. The technique described in this book has developed and evolved over the past three decades. The fundamentals and key steps discussed have been described as the "Safety Facelift". The aim of course is to avoid complications as much as possible. There are numerous techniques and procedures described and espoused at this time to improve facial appearance spanning a wide array from minimal approaches to very aggressive and invasive techniques. This spectrum is understandably confusing to the developing surgeon. It is not suggested that this text contains the only surgical answers and that other techniques are without merit. It is possible to state that the technique described herein will reliably provide appropriate results and help avoid serious complications.

The ultimate goal for this book is to provide a visually oriented text that in direct, easily understood, stepwise fashion provides the reader with a reliable, safe method for facelifts. Emphasis and importance is directed at careful patient analysis, selection of key and effective surgical steps, and avoidance of significant risk. Surgeons providing aesthetic facial changes create results that are visible and on display for all to appreciate or criticize. I hope that this text will contribute to surgical outcomes favorable to patients and surgeons alike.

J. Regan Thomas, MD

Table of Contents

1

Introduction: Facelift Rational and Procedural Alternatives

The facelift operation is well known both to the lay public as well as to physicians and surgeons. It is perhaps the procedure most associated with esthetic facial plastic surgery. Historically we have seen an evolution of the procedure, both in terms of technique as well in public acceptance and desirability. There was a period in the not-too-distant past that assumed individuals undergoing facelift were wealthy, celebrities, or in the entertainment business. Today, however, it is a generally excepted procedure and is explored by a wide spectrum of social, economic, and ethnic backgrounds. In part, that greater general acceptance has been due to enhanced safety and, hopefully, superior ultimate results. Similarly, no doubt it is coupled with an overall cultural desire for an enhanced self-perception of greater fitness and youth. Paralleling those desires is also a cultural pressure to maintain a youthful appearance related to work and economic environments in addition to various social interactions. Other terms describing the operation include rhytidectomy and, perhaps more appropriately, rhytidoplasty. Most surgeons and certainly the public at large, however, tend to use, understand, and appreciate the term "facelift." The title of this book as well as use of the term throughout the text will reflect this more common, perhaps better accepted term, facelift.[1]

The state of the art for the novice facial surgeon is a somewhat confusing array of procedures. No doubt the patient who explores these alternatives is also somewhat confused. Multiple facelift techniques and procedures are described in the literature and most have enthusiastic proponents and spokespersons. These procedures range from minimal surgical "minilifts," which are often described as being done under local anesthesia and as a brief outpatient visit even to the point of occasionally being termed "lunchtime procedures." At the other end of the spectrum are procedures that are significantly more invasive including the deep-plane procedures and composite facelift procedures. The so-called minilifts have unfortunately been popularized by the lay press and not infrequently provide less than ideal outcomes and only short-term improvements at best. These minilifts should be clearly differentiated from secondary and minimal incision facelifts, which, although more modest in their goals, may be part of a long-term treatment plan that enables the patient to have continued and highly effective improvement over long periods of time.

Variations of the deep-plane facelift including such alternatives as the extended subsuperficial muscular aponeurotic system (SMAS), the multiplane lift and the composite rhytidectomy have been well described.[2–5]

In general, the techniques have used deeper layers and dissect a sub-SMAS (as well as in certain anatomic regions, submuscular and subperiosteal) layer in an attempt to create greater improvement of facial foundation structures. Some authors feel that these deeper dissections enhance blood supply to the elevated soft tissues. This author has explored most of those procedures and concluded that these more invasive deeper layer procedures offered very

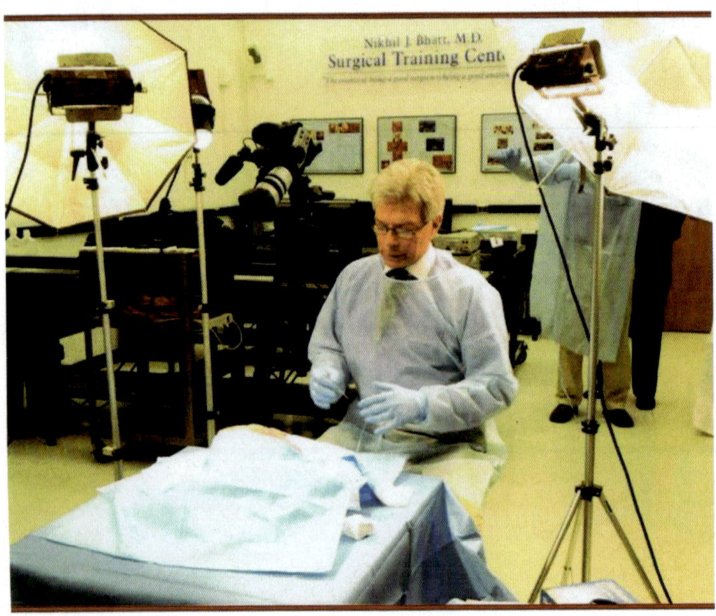

Figure 1-1. Precise anatomic dissection demonstrations will be used along with patient clinical photos to accurately demonstrate the "Safety Facelift".

little advantage in terms of the ultimate result for the patient[6].

These procedures potentially put the patient at greater risk for perioperative morbidity and possible complications. Many of these alternative procedures have been explored; the technique recommended here offers the best combination of safety with appropriate desirable results. Facelift is, of course, entirely elective in nature and so it seems prudent to expose the patient to as few risks as possible to achieve the ultimate goal. More aggressive surgical attempts to achieve an extraordinary result should be balanced with potential increased risk, as any complication, even if somewhat insignificant, represents a difficult conundrum when contemplating a totally elective procedure.

The technique described and illustrated in this text is a compilation of steps and procedures that have evolved over the past 30 years in the senior author's personal experience. Variations and alternative techniques have been explored and studied by the author with an eye toward achieving outstanding results for the patient while at the same time putting the patient at a minimum risk. The basics of this procedure have been published in other texts[1]; however, fine points and additional modifications have continued to evolve. This three-decade experience and genuine attempt to achieve appropriate results with a minimum of risk have resulted in what is often referred to as the "Safety Facelift."

The Safety Facelift

The facelift procedure necessarily entails a series of fundamental steps, including incision planning and placement, submental correction, flap elevation, SMAS, platysma, and deep-tissue tightening and repositioning, skin-flap repositioning, and tailoring and incision closure. From each of these fundamental steps the surgeon has available a variety of techniques and approaches, all of which have been well described in the literature. The Safety Facelift has evolved from looking at each of these fundamental steps and assessing which of the alternative techniques available will accomplish the intended result while at the same time create the least risk for potential complication. It is the compilation and assembly of these steps that together form the Safety Facelift procedure. The result is a procedure that provides both patient and surgeon the opportunity for an appropriate acceptable result with a minimum of risk for complication. Three decades of experience, trial and error, thoughtful study and exploration, and conscientious review follow-up and study are presented in the form of the technique presented here (**Figure 1-1**).

References

1. Tardy ME, Thomas, JR. *Facial Aesthetic Surgery*. St. Louis, Mosby-Yearbook, Inc., 1995.

2. Hamra ST. The deep plane rhytidectomy, *Plast Reconstr Surg*. 1992, 90, 1, 1–13.
3. Kamer FM. One hundred consecutive deep plane facelifts, *Arch* Otolaryngol Head Neck Surg. 1996, 122, 17–22.
4. Ramirez OM. The subperiosteal rhytidectomy: The third generation facelift. *Ann Plast Surg*. 1992, 28, 218–232.
5. Baker SR. Tri-plane rhytidectomy, *Arch Otolaryngol Head Neck Surg*. 1997, 123, 1167–1172.
6. Becker FF, Bassichis BA. Deep plane face-lift vs. SMAS plication face-lift, *Arch Facial Plast Surg*. 2004, 6, 8–13.

2

Facial Analysis and Preoperative Considerations

Surgical Candidate Selection

The most successful facelifts are typically in patients in whom the aging process has been less severe, are minimally obese, and can benefit from what is often described as good bone structure. Changes in facial appearance over time are often the result of diverse factors including genetic predisposition, actinic and sun damage, potential stress, and other influences that are collectively perceived as aging[1,2]. Chronologic age is an unreliable determinate because these factors, coupled with the patient's own self-image and perception, create the need for potential surgery within a wide spectrum of time **(Figures 2-1 and 2-2)**. As in all aesthetic procedures the patient must have realistic expectations in order to make rational decisions regarding surgery. An insightful psychological evaluation of the patient, their expectations, and potential for acceptance of realistic results are all an important part of an initial patient evaluation. Patients who do not possess these attributes are not candidates for elective aesthetic surgery.

Ideal physical characteristics for a facelift from an anatomic standpoint might well be described as an attractive healthy female patient typically beyond the age of 40. In a general sense, males are often poor candidates because of heavier, thicker hair-bearing skin and soft tissues (and perhaps more frequently challenging psychological issues). Skin characteristics ideally should include remnants of appropriate elasticity with a lack of actinic solar and other environmental skin damage. The obese patient with heavy deposits of adipose fat in the cheek, jawline, and submental cervical areas are increasingly a less favorable candidate as the magnitude of adipose content increases. The best facial skeleton is one that is strong, angular, and attractively developed particularly in the mandibular and malar regions. A strong chinline significantly increases the likelihood of good results and at times may require surgical chin augmentation to accomplish that goal. A high cervical angle with high positioning of the hyoid and thyroid complex again allows for superior results in the lower face and neck region. Relative anatomic issues including submaxillary gland ptosis and a short, wide neck or hypertrophied musculature also take away from ideal results for rejuvenation surgery.

Obese patients should be counseled that their results are going to be limited and their expectations should be lowered. These patients are best counseled to plan on a realistic weight loss program prior to pursuing surgery. Indeed, patients who are actively trying to lose weight should be counseled to obtain a stable weight prior to surgery. Weight loss after surgery will potentially allow for laxity of the tissue. Certainly, the patient should understand that facelift itself, including some strategic liposuction, is not a weight reduction procedure. Similarly, patients with premature loss of elasticity of facial skin, either from

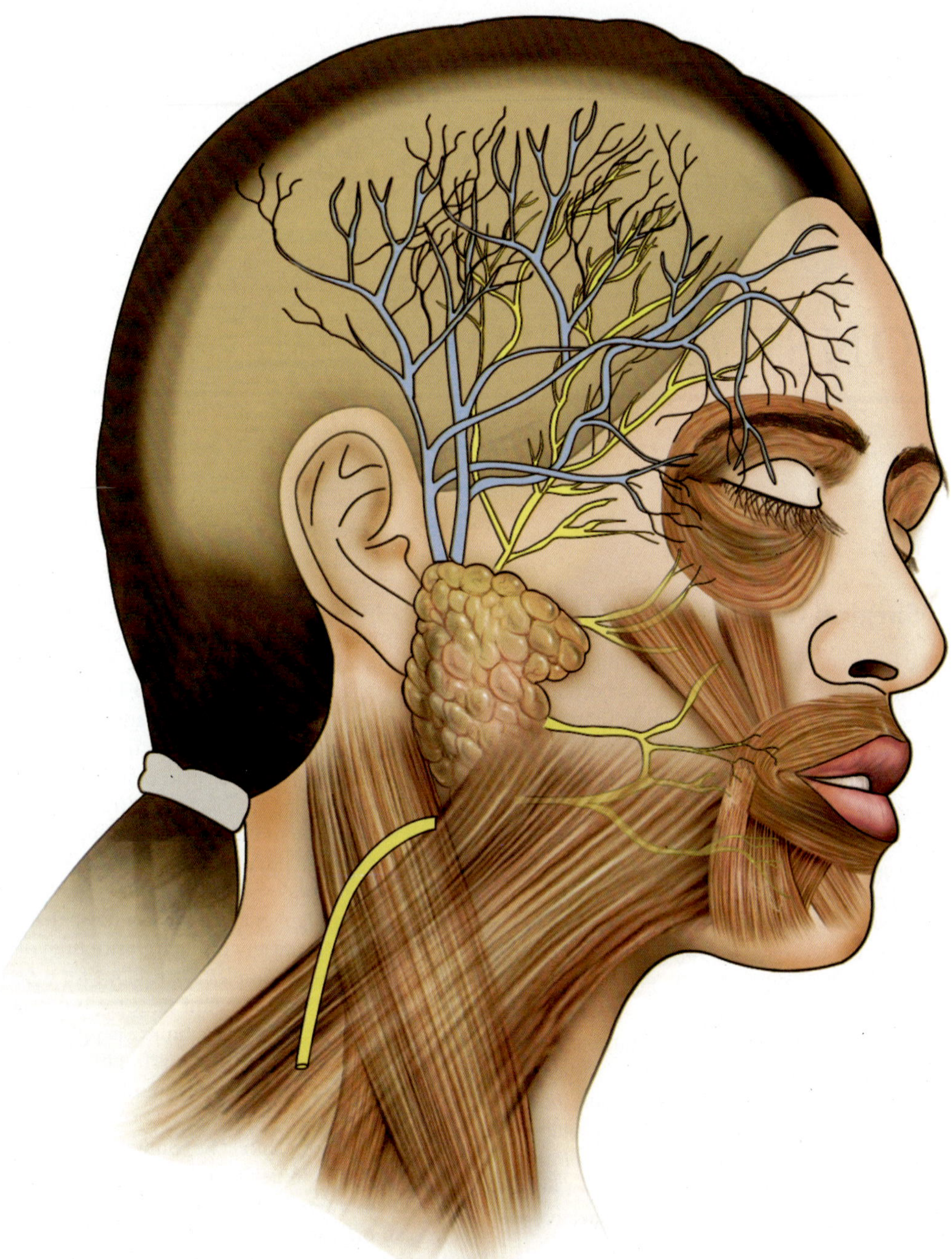

Figure 2-1. Pertinent facial-cervical anatomy for facelift. Safety Facelift avoids potential injury to key structures.

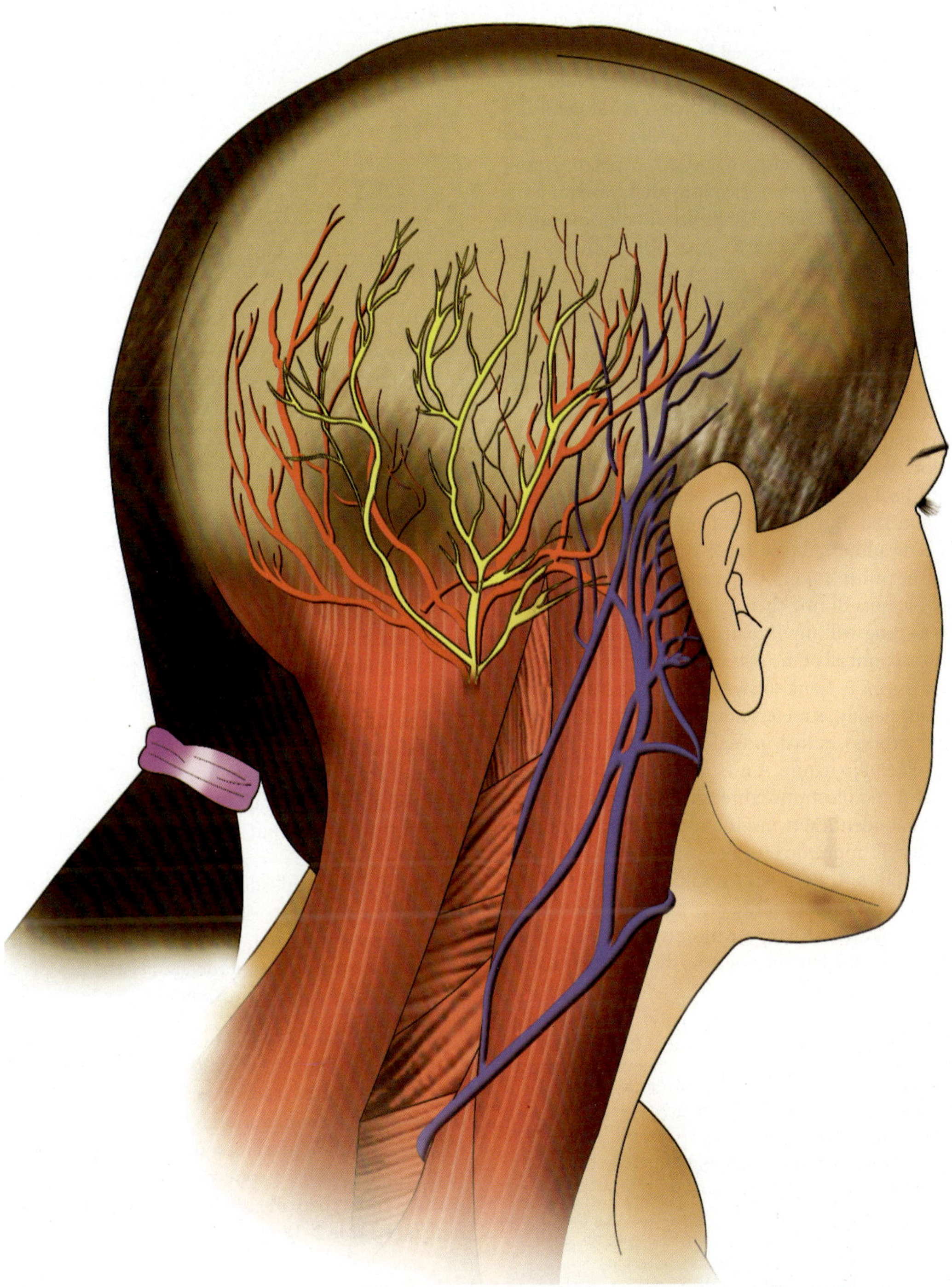

Figure 2-2. Postauricular and occipital anatomy.

hereditary factors or from sun damage, will have a less satisfactory prolongation and duration of improvement as well as initial limitations.

Due to the elective nature of this procedure, ideal candidates also should have no systemic or other complicating factors related to their ability to safely undergo surgery and avoid postoperative complications. Any medications that have an anticoagulant effect including aspirin and nonsteroidal anti-inflammatory drugs should be stopped. Prescription medications that may affect this issue should be coordinated with the patient's personal physician to avoid postoperative bleeding, ecchymoses, and potential hematoma. Smoking is a significant issue for facelift patients and the surgeon should insist the patient stop smoking completely and maintain that abstinence at least 3-6 months prior to surgery. Frank discussions about difficulties with healing and potential for infection and scarring in the smoking patient should be frankly and directly addressed (**see Table 2-1**).

The most common question asked by potential patients during their initial facelift interview is: "how long will my facelift last?" The answer takes into account all of the issues noted previously in this discussion. A frank answer, which points out that because aging is a constant, progressive and inevitable process, is that indeed the facelift will not be permanent in nature. A useful analogy that has been helpful and illustrative through the years is to compare two identical twins. If one twin has a facelift he or she will appear to be more youthful than the twin who does not. Both will continue to age in subsequent years; however, the one who had the facelift will always tend to appear more youthful and with fewer changes than the one who did not. This seems to be a realistic and useful description that most patients can understand. Similarly, it is noted to the patients they may require secondary "tuck-up" or ancillary procedures at periods depending on the nature of their soft tissue and their on going lifestyle. Many patients appreciate the concept of "preventative maintenance" as an approach to maintaining their best possible appearance (**see Table 2-2**).

TABLE 2-1 Selection of the Ideal Patient

1. Healthy patient without systemic disease whose facial-cervical skin and muscle appear excessive, redundant, and ptotic.
2. Facial appearance characterized by strong angular bony skeleton with a normal or high-positioned hyoid–thyroid complex.
3. Patient at or near ideal weight possessing minimal facial fat with retained facial skin elasticity.
4. Patient without deeply wrinkled, creased, or actinically damaged skin.
5. A realistic and motivated patient where the goals of surgery are for improvement and not perfection. The patient understands anatomical and technical limitations of the purposed surgery.

TABLE 2-2 Poor Patient Characteristics

1. Systemic health issues including diabetes, vascular abnormalities, conditions requiring anticoagulants, or patients who smoke.
2. Facial obesity and adipose excess.
3. Poor chin projection, a low hyoid thyroid complex with poor cervical middle angle.
4. Ptotic submandibular glands.
5. Deep nasolabial or melolabial grooves and creases.
6. Patients with unrealistic expectations and goals.

In summary, the ideal patient for facelift surgery includes the following:

1. A healthy patient whose facial and cervical skin and soft tissues are redundant ptotic and no longer conform in a youthful manner to the bony skeleton.
2. Facial anatomy that is characterized by a strong angular bony skeleton with a normally positioned hyoid and thyroid cartilage complex.
3. Ideal weight without excess facial or submental fat.
4. Minimally actinically damaged skin without deeply wrinkled creases or rhytid-laden skin.
5. A highly motivated patient who has realistic goals for surgery and understands and accepts a realistic degree of improvement.

No degree of surgical skill can compensate for a poorly selected patient. Even the patient who is appropriately selected from an anatomic aspect will be disappointed if an operation is being done for inappropriate psychological reasons and goals on behalf of the patient. These concepts are true for facelift perhaps more than any other aesthetic facial procedure (**see Table 2-3**).

Anesthesia Considerations

To some degree, the decision as to the type of anesthesia to be selected for a facelift procedure is based on a combination of the patient's desires coupled with the preferences of the surgeon in a general

TABLE 2-3 Possible Signs of the "Difficult Patient"

1. Recent life trauma (divorce, job loss, death of loved one).
2. Numerous previous aesthetic procedures (especially if unhappy results).
3. Minimal or imperceptible clinical problem about which the patient is concerned.
4. History of significant psychological problems or personality disorders.
5. Difficult or unusual behavior with the physician or the staff.

sense as well as specifically for that patient. Because of the frequent exposure to the public by various proponents of "minilifts" and minimal approach facelift procedures through marketing endeavors and the lay press, patients may have the concept of all facelift procedures can be done using local anesthesia. At the other end of the spectrum, a great many patients are concerned about the possibility of discomfort during the procedure or have a sense of nervousness related to being in the operating room environment. A thorough discussion preoperatively about the alternatives as well as the surgeon's preference should be shared with the patient and one should ensure that the patient has a good understanding of the pros and cons of this selection. The rationale for selection of anesthesia, in addition to a frank discussion regarding safety issues, should be part of the preoperative consultation.

Most genuine facelift operations including the Safety Facelift would be difficult to accomplish with appropriate patient comfort through local anesthesia alone. Once this is explained to the patient, it would be unusual for the patient to want to pursue one of the other alternatives.

Local anesthesia plus intravenous sedation is an alternative that is comfortable for many surgeons. Certainly the patient can be made quite comfortable throughout the case with this approach. A MAC anesthesia approach (monitored anesthesia control), if done expertly and in an appropriate environment, is certainly an approach to anesthesia that lends itself to the operation and one that maintains a comfortable patient. There are fundamental and key requirements if this approach is to be used. First is an experienced anesthesiologist who is properly monitoring the patient for a procedure that may require several hours. An adequate airway with good oxygenation is mandatory as is appropriate monitoring equipment for oxygenation levels of the patient throughout the entire case. Preparation, instrumentation, and expertise should be immediately available at all times should the patient require intubation. The same preparation environment and expertise should be available for the patient who is having sedation anesthesia in exactly the same manner as though general anesthesia was going to be used.

The author typically uses endotracheal intubation and general anesthesia for nearly all facelift patients. Exceptions are made for patients who need a relatively small amount of preparation and perhaps a shorter time expectation for the procedure. This would be true for the secondary tuck-up type of procedure as well. However, experience has shown that most patients are significantly more comfortable having a general endotracheal anesthesia with modern anesthesia agents and expert care from the anesthesiologist. These patients do well and typically maintain a comfortable postoperative experience. Most importantly, however, is the enhanced safety of having a patient with a controlled airway maintaining appropriate oxygenation. Most life-threatening events reported relating to facelift surgery have been related to airway issues and improper oxygenation of the patient leading to secondary complications. Nearly all patients understand and agree with use of general anesthesia once they have an appropriate and realistic understanding of the safety issues coupled with the ensuring of their comfort during the procedure and perioperative time period (**see Table 2-4**).

TABLE 2-4 Anesthesia Considerations

1. Most patients for facelift benefit from general anesthesia with an endotracheal controlled airway.
2. All patients should have appropriate monitoring including fully monitored observation for blood pressure, oxygen saturation, and cardiac function.
3. Local infiltration of lidocaine with epinephrine is useful to both allow good anesthesia and maximum hemostasis from vasoconstriction.
4. Usually 1% lidocaine with 1:100,000 epinephrine is used. Volume of lidocaine is minimized through stepwise injection of the areas to be infiltrated and postponing subsequent injection to other areas until that regions has had its surgery completed. Sequential infiltration performed 10–15 minutes prior to incisions on the subsequent side is safe and effective.

References

1. Larabee WF, Makielski KH, Henderson JL. *Surgical Anatomy of the Face*. Philadelphia, Lippincott Williams and Wilkins, 2004.
2. Zimbler, Thomas JR, Pretreatment with botulinum A toxin improves laser resurfacing results: A prospective randomized blinded trial, *Arch Facial Plast Surg*. 3 (3), 2001 165–169.

3

Surgical Technique

Preoperative Preparation

Patients are asked to shampoo their hair and wash their faces, removing all makeup and other grooming products the evening before and the morning of surgery.

In the preoperative holding area, with the patient awake and in the upright and animated position, areas of attention are marked with a surgical marking pen. This includes the location of jowl laxity, submental fat, and platysmal banding. Appropriate marks for other secondary procedures that are also being performed at the same as the facelift are similarly marked. The incision location within the hairline is marked and the hair is controlled through twist-tie bunching of hair segments in small elastic bands. No hair around the incision is trimmed or shaved.

Once in the operating room, and following intubation by the anesthesiologist, all appropriate surgical preparations by the operating room staff are performed. The patient's head is positioned superiorly to the upper edge of the operating table.

Incision sites and areas to be undermined are then injected with 1% lidocaine with 1:100,000 epinephrine local anesthetic (**Figure 3-1a**). Each region is sequentially injected prior to surgical

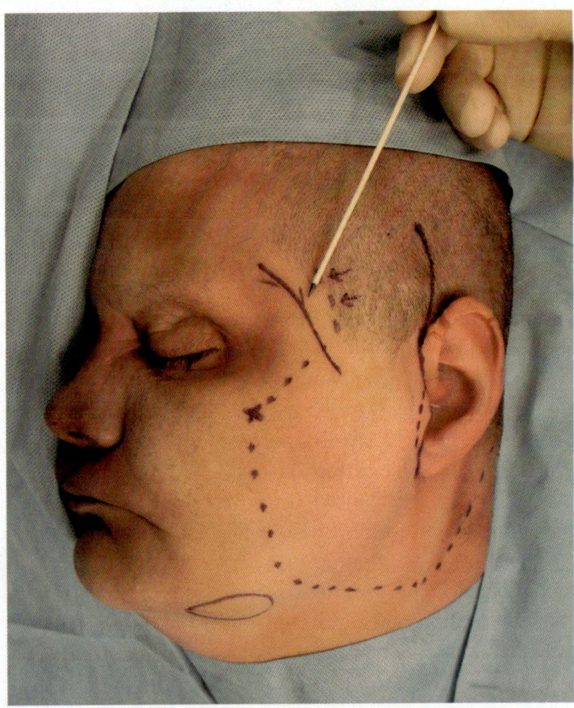

Figure 3-1a. Cadaver example of typical incision sites, extent of undermining and the course of the temporal branch of facial nerve.

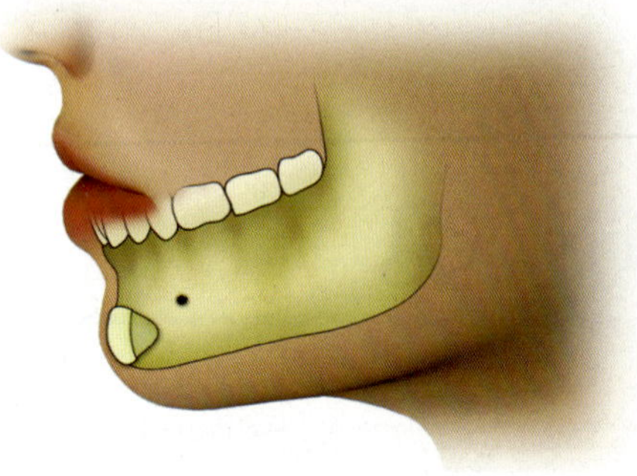

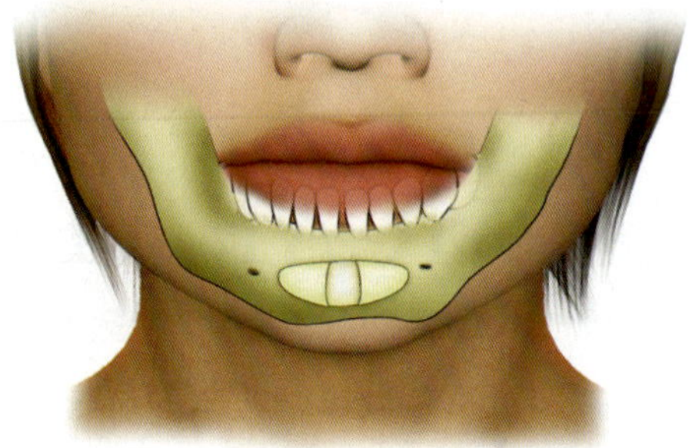

Figure 3-1b. Placement of chin implants in patient population with a degree of retrognathia or poor chin projection.

attention to that region, which allows the initial and previous injections to be safely metabolized. The usual steps sequentially include initial submental correction, followed by the first side of the face and finishing with the second side. This sequential injection acts both as a safety measure for the patient, avoiding an excessive epinephrine effect as well as maintaining appropriate physiologic levels of the local anesthetic.

The patient is then prepped and draped in the usual fashion and the endotracheal tube is usually sterilely draped separately so that it is visible throughout the procedure and can be moved and positioned as required. A sterile cotton ball, which has been saturated in an antiseptic solution, is typically placed in the external auditory canal bilaterally to avoid blood or other drainage to accumulate in the external canal. This also seals off an area of potential contamination knowing that the areas of the canal may not have been prepped as aggressively as other areas of the face and neck.

Submental Correction

Typically, the first step in the facelift addresses the submental area. This will include removing excess adipose through liposuction, correcting and plicating submental platysmal bands as required, and potentially excising a small amount of submental redundant skin. The correction of the submental region allows for enhanced improvement of the cervical angle and forms a basis for which the lateral elevation repositioning and support can be accomplished[1]. The area to be addressed in the submental region, jowl area, and platysmal bands have been marked when the patient was in the preoperative area in the upright animated position. Incision position and the submental crease have also been marked. After introduction of anesthesia and prior to prepping, the area has been infiltrated with 1% lidocaine with 1:100,000 epinephrine. If there is a previous scar from earlier surgery, or perhaps trauma, this can be incorporated as part of the incision. In the patient population that has a degree of retrognathia or poor chin projection (**Figure 3-1b**) the results can be enhanced by placement of chin implant **Table 3-1**).

Augmentation of the chin through an implant is accomplished through the submental incision and can be done during this major step of the facelift procedure (**Figure 3-2**). An implant is placed in a subperiosteal pocket that has been formed with a periosteal elevator. A central strip of periosteum is left intact to help avoid bony erosion from the implant material. In essence then there is a central area of periosteum against which the implant is positioned and the lateral ends of the implant are placed within a subperiosteal pocket which is carefully created so that there is a precise fit for the implant. This precise positioning avoids mobility and movement of the implant. The implant is further secured by suture placement securing the implant to the periosteum of the central portion of the chin.

Although not all patients will require that removal of fat and platysmal plication, many do. In individuals with minimal adipose in the submental area and no visible platysmal bands, this step may be omitted; however, that is an unusual situation in the majority of facelift patients. Some attention to

TABLE 3-1 Chin Implant Enhancements

1. Improved chin projection.
2. Enhanced cervicomental angle.
3. Better repositioning of soft-tissue rectors.
4. Balance facial relationships and proportions.

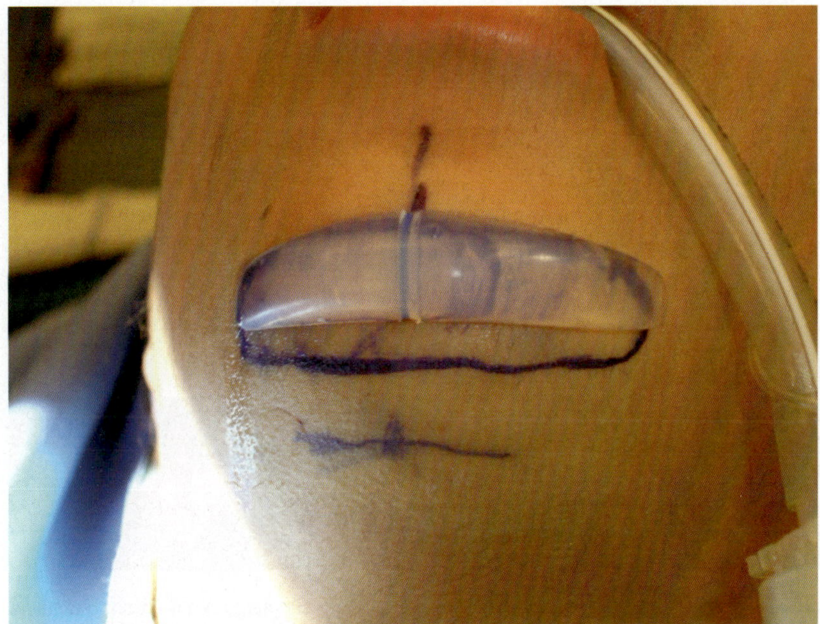

Figure 3-2. A solid silicone rubber chin implant may be placed through the submental incision to enhance chin projection.

the submandibular jowl regions is also frequently required.

Removing adipose tissue is accomplished through liposuction[2]. An initial small (less that 1 cm) incision is made in the chin at the submental crease (**see Figure 3-3**). This small incision allows for placement of liposuction cannulas (**Figures 3-4 and 3-5**) while helping to maintain appropriate negative pressure

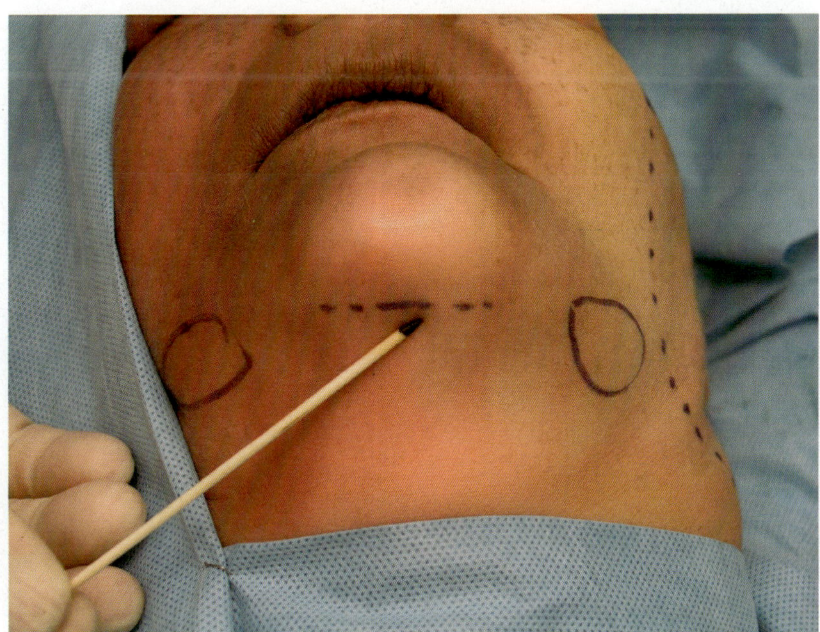

Figure 3-3. Incision position in the submental crease is marked in the preoperative session.

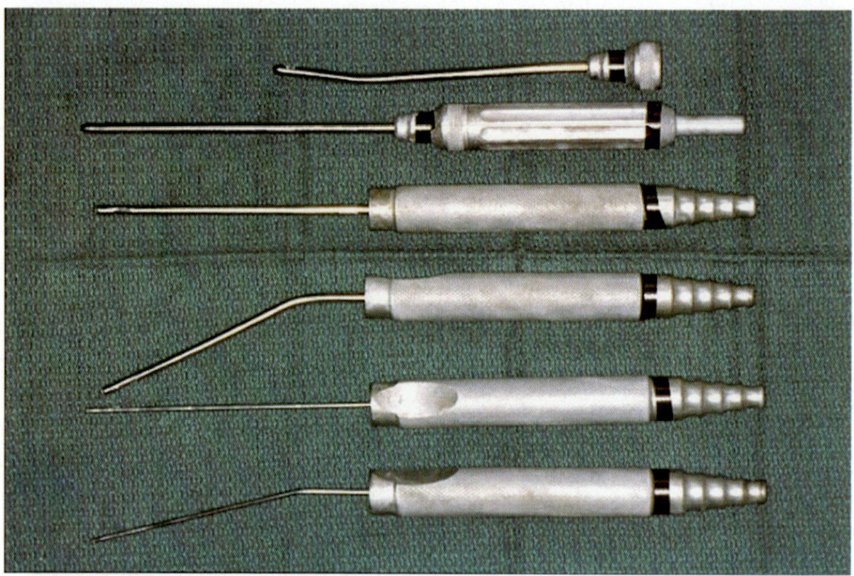

Figure 3-4. A variety of cannula shapes are available for submental liposuction. Usually a 2- and 4-mm cannula are ideal.

at the same time. Through that initial incision using small scissors and forceps, a subcutaneous plane is developed a short distance to help maintain the proper layer for fat removal (**Figure 3-6**). Multiple small tunnels are then created with a 2 or 3 mm liposuction cannula. No suction is applied initially, creating small tunnels through the submental incision throughout the submental area to the cervical angle and extending into the jowl region below the mandible bilaterally. The lateral borders of this submental liposuction maneuver will be the anterior borders of the sternoclavicular mastoid muscles

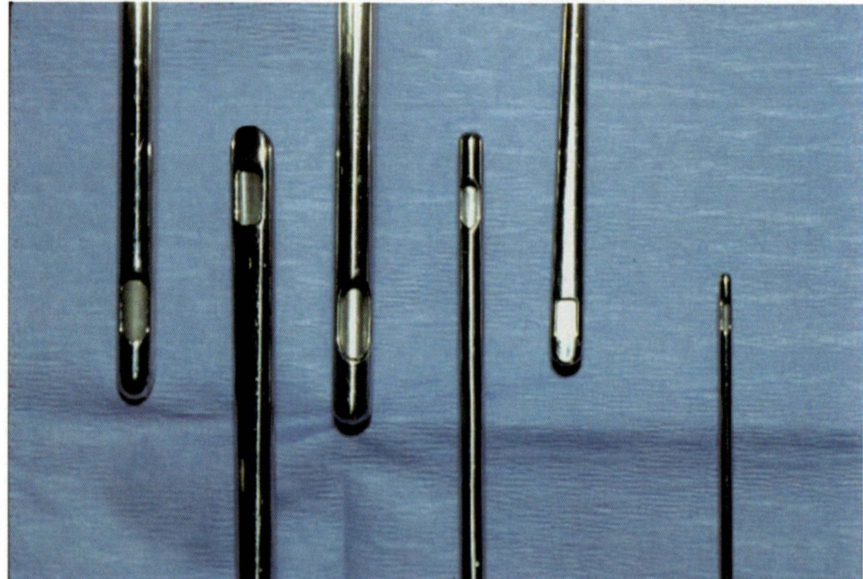

Figure 3-5. Cannula tips should be selected that have a single suction hole for greater accuracy.

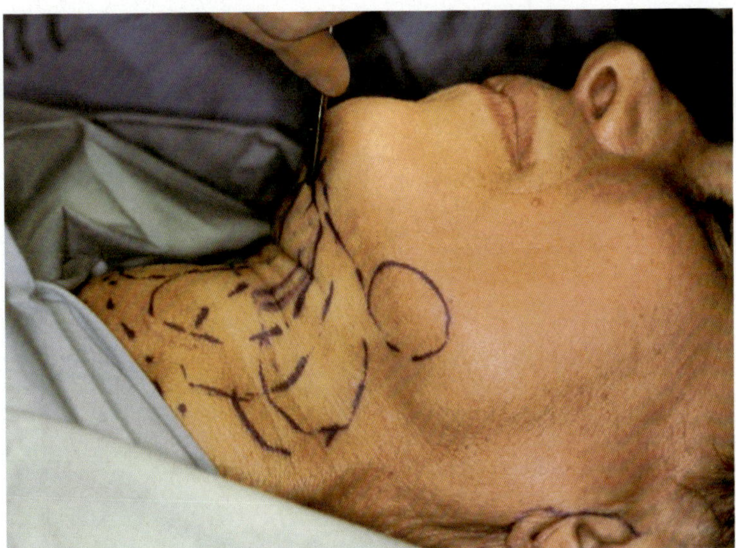

Figure 3-6. A subcutaneous plane is developed a short distance to ensure that the proper plane is established.

laterally and the cervical angle inferiorly. Using the 2 or 3 mm cannula, tunnels are created in a fanlike fashion across the neck from one mandibular area to the other (**Figure 3-7**). A 4-mm cannula is now placed with active suction created using the preformed tunnels for ease of passage of the cannula itself. The back and forth, to and fro maneuvers are utilized to gently suction fat away from the submental area (**Figure 3-8**). Great care is taken to ensure that the openings of the cannula are away from the skin and dermis and toward the fat to prevent any groovelike affect on the under surface of the skin flap that is being developed. This is facilitated by using a cannula that has a hole only on one side so that the other side, which is against the dermis, does not create suction. It is often helpful to use a spatula or flattened tip for the 4-mm cannula to effect greater ease of fat removal and contouring. Manual manipulation is used throughout this maneuver with the opposite hand gently rolling fat and soft tissue into the path of the cannula as it is being maneuvered in the fanlike fashion in the submental area. When suctioning in the jowl region, it is critical to avoid using the mandible margin as a fulcrum or to place pressure on the mandible, which could create a pressure injury to the marginal mandibular nerve.

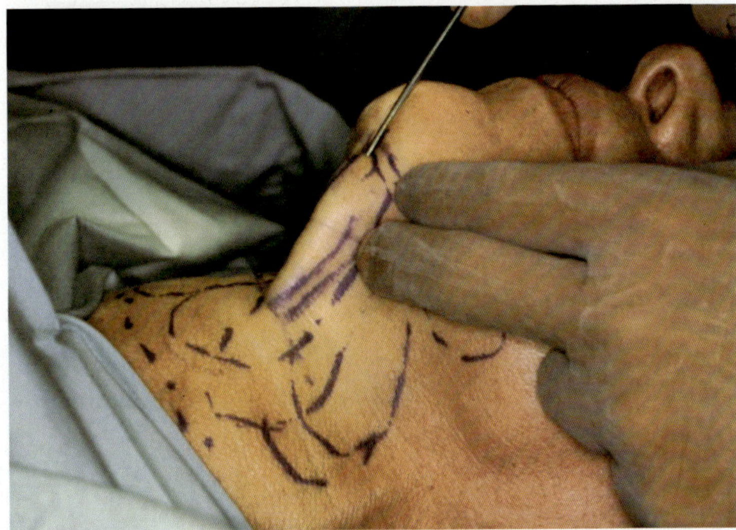

Figure 3-7. A 2-mm cannula is used to create initial subcutaneous tunnels.

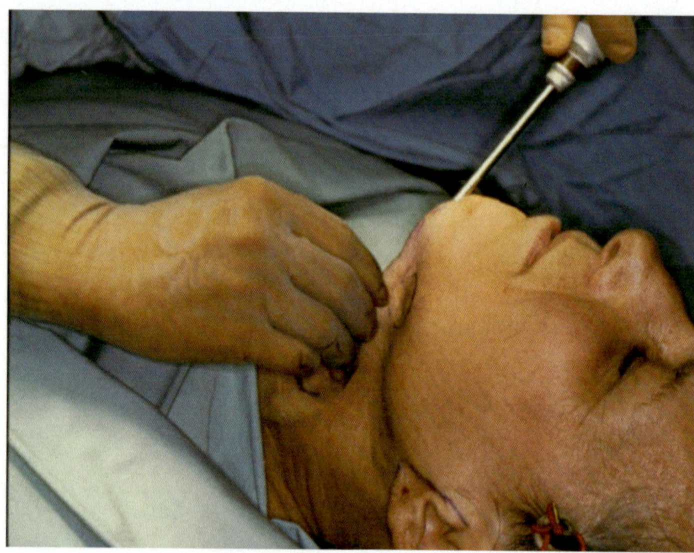

Figure 3-8. Liposuction is accomplished with the hole of the cannula toward the fat and away from the dermis.

Experience has shown that removing adipose through liposuction is less likely to create an over-resection of fat and a so-called cobralike hollowness in the submental area. This is a sign of overresection of the fat and should be avoided. Liposuction allows for better contouring and feathering laterally and avoidance of overresection in the central region. In addition to fat being removed from the subcutaneous layer, subplatysmal fat occasionally needs to be resected but should be done very carefully and judiciously. Most often, fat removal is confined to the subcutaneous region. Upon completion of liposuction in all regions, the patient is examined and the soft tissue is palpated to help ensure appropriate adipose removal in addition to symmetry.

Following completion of removal of submental fat, a decision is required as to whether the submental area needs further enhancement through tightening of the platysma muscle. Certainly, those patients who have visible platysma bands preoperatively require this step. At this point, the submental incision is extended to $2\frac{1}{2}$ to 3 cm in length (**Figure 3-9**). This is typically curvilinear to avoid extension of the incision to the margin of the mandible on either side where it might be visible. This incision allows for visibility of the submental area

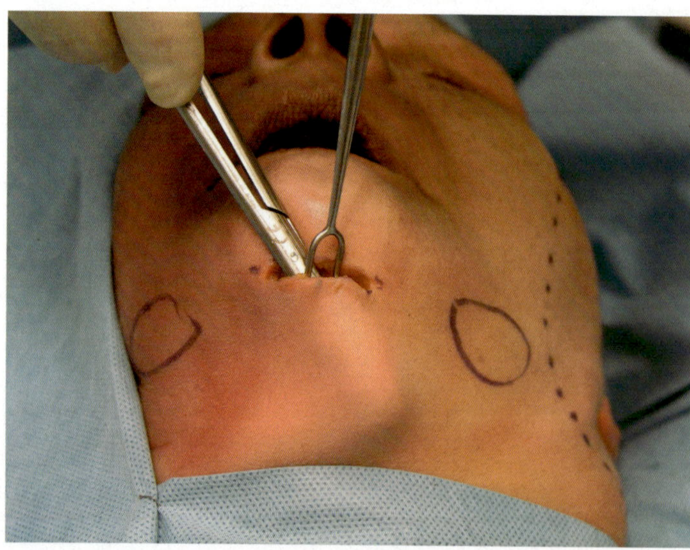

Figure 3-9. Following liposuction the submental flap is undermined to reveal the platysma muscles.

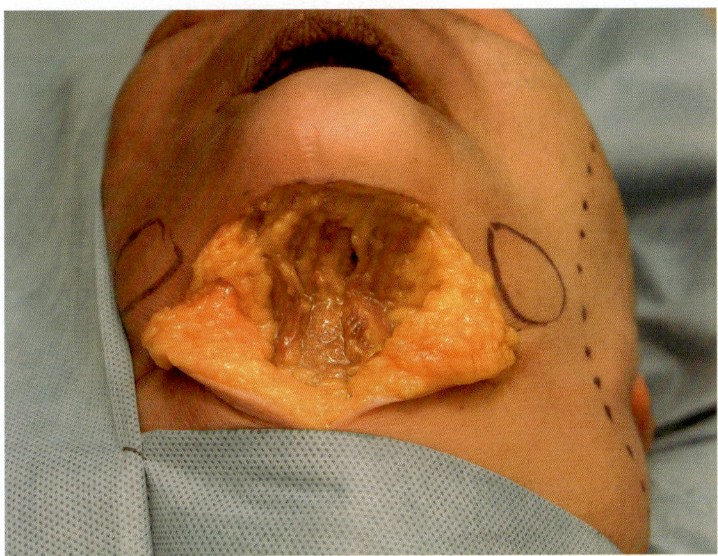

Figure 3-10. A cadaver preparation demonstrates the skin reflected to view platysmal muscle edges.

including the medial margins of the platysmal muscles. These medial margins if redundant or lax are visible clinically as platysmal bands (**Figures 3-10 and 3-11**).

A submental flap is then created by connecting the liposuction tunnels. This is usually easily accomplished in a bloodless fashion. The medial platysmal edges are identified and platysmal muscle is visible laterally from the central neck (**see Figure 3-12**). The platysmal margins are now grasped and a subplatysmal plane is elevated with scissor spreading. Effectively bilateral platysmal muscle flaps have been created, and hemostasis is maintained with bipolar cautery throughout this step. Next, the level the cervical angle is determined and corresponds to preoperative external markings. At this point a 2-cm

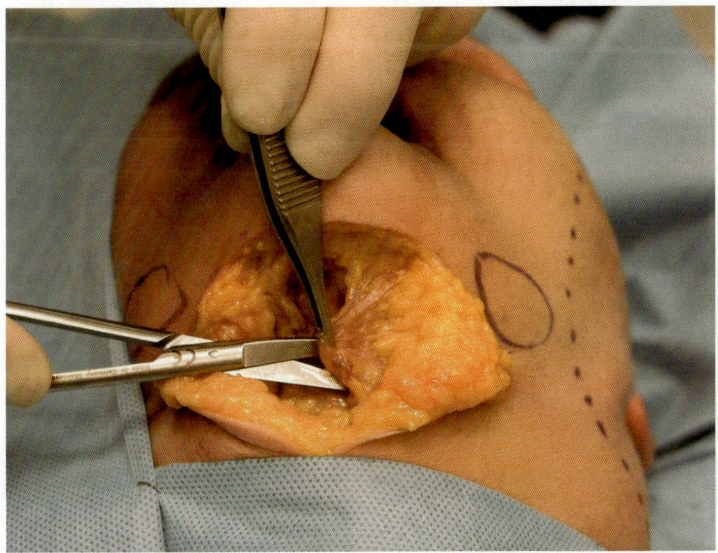

Figure 3-11. A cadaver demonstration of undermining platysmal margins prior to advancement and plication.

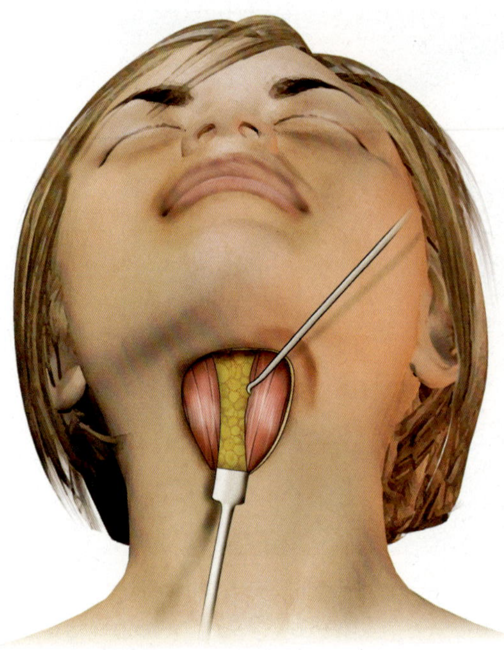

Figure 3-12. Following submental liposuction, the medial platysmal margins are identified.

(**Figure 3-13**) horizontal incision is made through the platysmal muscle following cautery by bipolar cautery tips. As required, bipolar cautery is effective for any bleeding points (**Figure 3-14**). Dividing the vertical bands of muscle in this fashion allows for creation of the cervical angle in addition to facilitating advancement and plication of the more anterior platysmal edges superiorly. This division of the platysma is referred to as breaking up the "verticality" of the platysmal bands. If one thinks

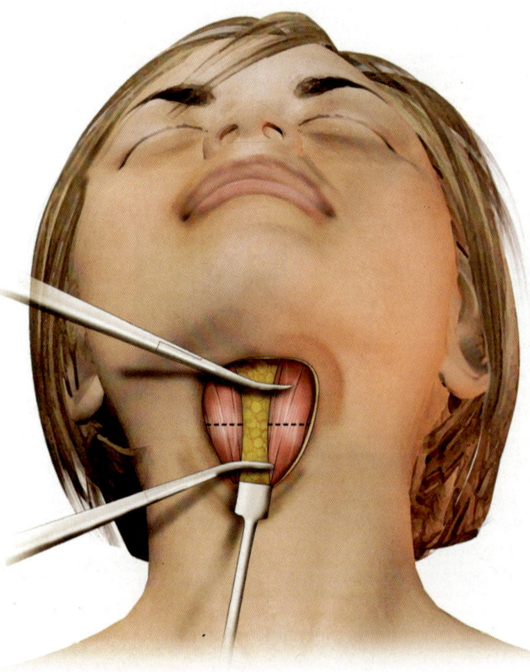

Figure 3-13. A horizontal incision at the level corresponding to the cervical angle is created 2 cm long.

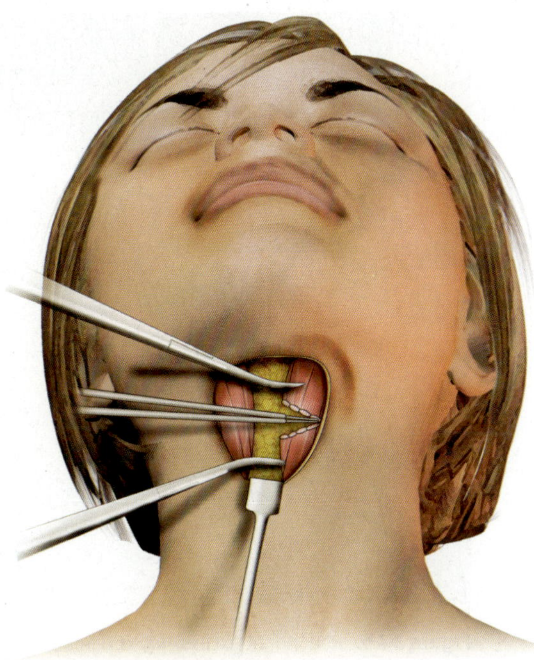

Figure 3-14. Muscle edges are cauterized with bipolar cautery.

of the platysmal bands being a vertical line from the submental area through the cervical angle, the horizontal incision breaks up that vertical line and allows for further tightening of the submental region. Occasionally, there is so much redundancy of the platysma that the medial margins can be excised conservatively. The medial edges are then advanced anterior to the horizontal incision and sutured together with an absorbable 4-0 polydioxanone sutures **(Figure 3-15).** This effectively tightens the submental neck and restores a more youthful cervical angle by creating a supportive sling effect. This

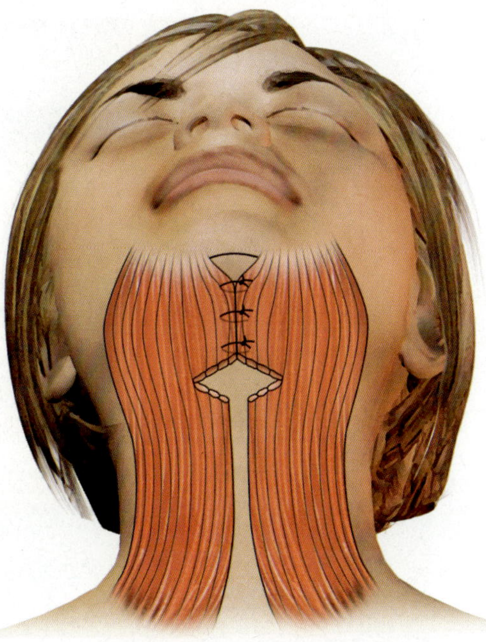

Figure 3-15. Medial edges of the platysma muscle are advanced and sutured together with H-polydioxanone sutures.

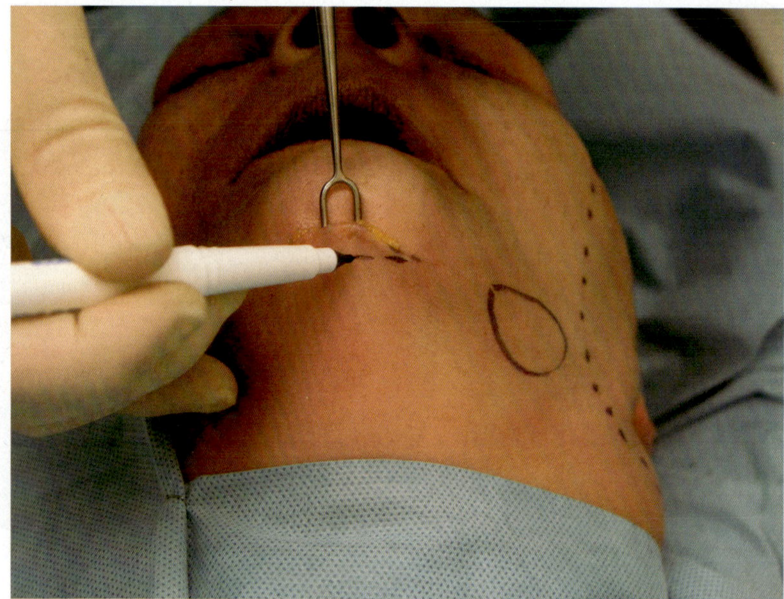

Figure 3-16. Redundant excess skin is demarcated and excised.

is often referred to as a platysmal corset maneuver. The skin is now redraped over the new anatomic foundation. A small amount of redundant or excess skin can be excised at this point. Because there is no tension on the wound, typically this incision is closed in a single layer with interrupted 6-0 polypropylene sutures. Precise hemostasis is obtained through-out the procedure with bipolar cautery and there is no need for a drain routinely (**Figures 3-16 and 3-17**).

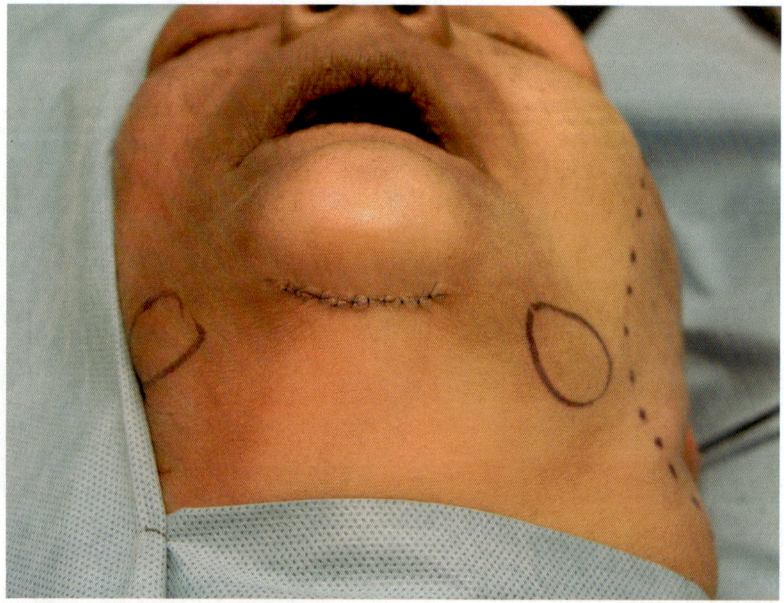

Figure 3-17. Closure of the submental incision without tension.

Facial Incisions

Selection of incision placement is critical to obtaining superior results in facelift surgery. In addition to giving access to the deep planes as well as undermining and resecting the loose and redundant skin and soft tissue, incision placement has an obvious direct relationship to the visibility (more importantly lack of visibility) of the scars. This is of key importance to the patient, understandably. Incisional scar visibility makes a difference between a successful result and a less than optimal postoperative appearance. Incision planning is based to some degree on physician preference and a variety of incision designs are described in the literature. It is perhaps more important to develop incision design and placement based on the patients specific anatomy including hairline position and to adapt the most inconspicuous and yet utilitarian incision for that specific individual.[3]

In the temporal area, it is important to hide the incision, give access to the upper portion of the facelift procedure, and avoid visible shifting of the hairline or temporal hair tuft region. It is preferable to avoid pretrichial incisions. Although these incisions have potential advantage of avoiding a hair tuft shift, the obvious risk of a visible scar is always present. A curvilinear incision starting a variable distance above the ear in the temporal area has proven to be superior in most situations. (**Figure 3-18**). This allows elevation of subfollicular plane of the hair-bearing skin and appropriately hides the scar. It is felt that a curved incision rather than a straight vertical incision helps to interrupt the forces of contracture while maintaining an appropriate incision and avoids significant shift of the hairline. Most frequently, this incision begins 2–4 cm above the superior helix within the temporal area and is carried slightly posterior and downward with a gently curved C configuration. Variation on this design is at times needed in situations where the hairline temple tuft is congenitally high or perhaps has been elevated from previous surgery (**Figure 3-19**). In this situation, further elevation would be undesirable and modification of the incision is used. The inferior portion of the incision at the preauricular superior helix is curved anteriorly in this situation, creating a subtle S-shape configuration that preserves hair-bearing soft tissue in its preoperative state at this preauricular junction. This allows upper lifting of the face without significantly displacing the preauricular hair tuft or sideburn hair. Again, it should be stressed that experience has shown that it is preferable to avoid prehairline incisions in the temporal region.

In the preauricular portion of the procedure, there are, again, various alternatives for incision placement. Most often the patient benefits from an

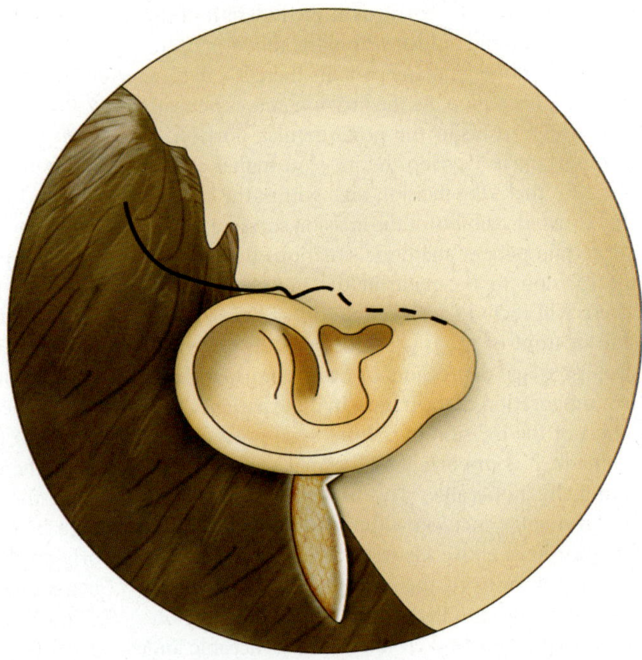

Figure 3-18. The temporal incision is hidden within the hairline and creates a curvilinear configuration above the ear.

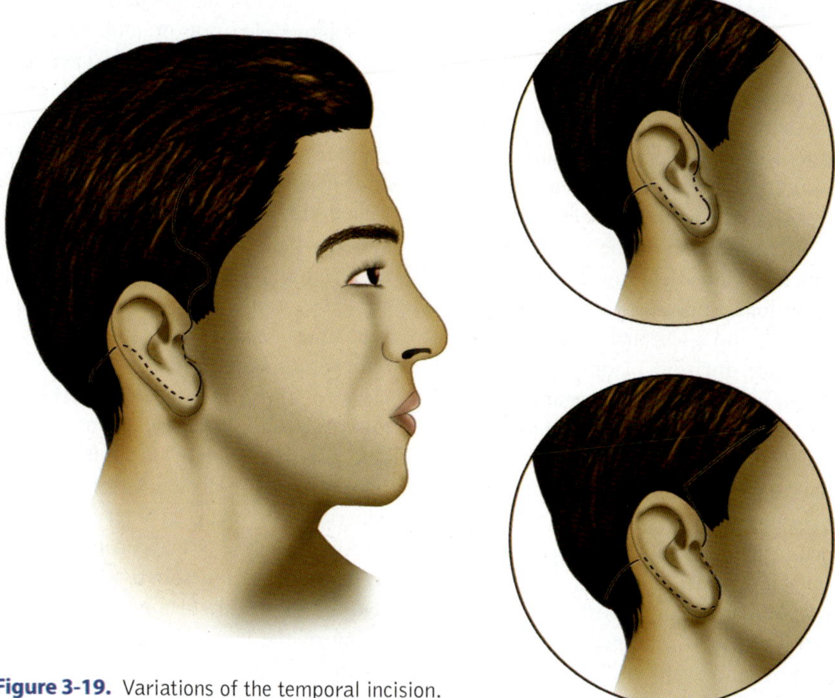

Figure 3-19. Variations of the temporal incision.

incision that moves the scar away from the preauricular region and hides the incision just posterior to the edge of the tragus. This, in effect, develops an incision that is hidden within the ear and avoids a preauricular sign of surgery. The incision exits at the inferior edge of the tragus at the junction of the earlobe tissue and hidden within the junction of the cheek to earlobe. In many patients there is a natural crease in this region. As the incision curves beneath the earlobe to begin the postauricular portion, is it important to develop the incision higher at this point to "tuck" the incision high within the earlobe cleft to avoid visibility of the incision scar line. There are certain patient anatomic situations that require the incision to be made in the pretragal region. These will include a patient who has hair-bearing skin in front of the tragus, possesses an extremely deep pretragal depression, or has an unusual shape or configuration of the tragus. In these patients, variation of the incision in the pretragal position can be made. It is important still to make this incision minimally noticeable. This is best accomplished by curving the incision within the incisura and the superior helix above the tragus and then a secondary curvature from the incisura back anterior to the tragus and into the preauricular earlobe region. This irregular or broken line is less noticeable and better camouflaged than a straight incision in most female patients who cannot otherwise use a posttragal incision.

In the male patient, the presence of hair-bearing skin in the midface region also requires modification of the incision. This facial beard or hair-bearing skin would not be appropriate to move to the posttragal area, and therefore the incision is placed in a single skin crease anterior to the tragus extends inferiorly to the earlobe region **(Figure 3-20)**. The temporal incision in the male patient does not extend as high and is curved anteriorly to preserve the sideburn. The remaining portion of the incision in the male patient is the same as in the female patient. The male patient should be advised that because of shifting and elevation of the skin that indeed the hair-bearing portion of facial skin may be shifted and that in some individuals shaving patterns may need to be altered including shaving beneath or even posterior to the earlobe.

In the postauricular area, the incision continues from the junction with the preauricular incision high beneath the earlobe cleft and extends superiorly on the posterior concha by 3–5 mm. To some it may seen counterintuitive not to hide the incision within the postauricular sulcus itself. However, experience has shown that this incision tends to

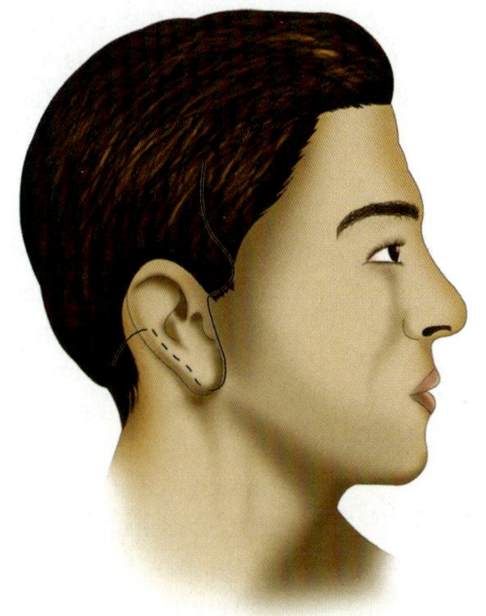

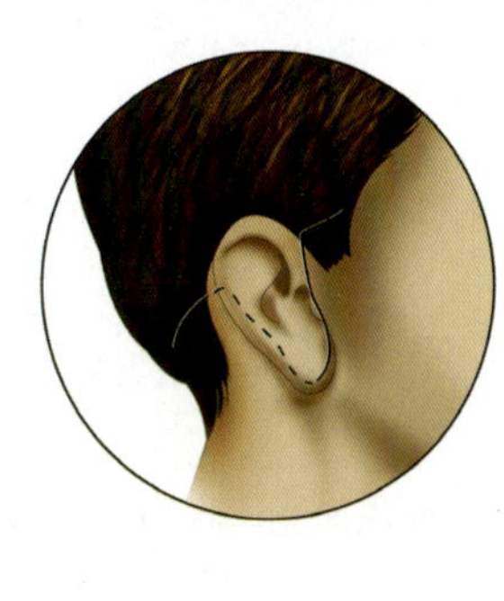

Figure 3-20. Incision in the male patient is modified and designed to avoid advancing bearded skin or to the tragus or shift sideburn hair.

shift following closure of the postauricular flap. If the incision is placed within the sulcus it moves away from the sulcus and potentially is more visible. To the contrary, an incision that has been placed on the concha typically shifts to the sulcus, preserving an inconspicuous position (**Figure 3-21**).

The incision continues superiorly to a level typically just above a point that would correspond to the height of the superior portion of the external auditory canal. Depending on hair position, and the position of the auricle itself, this may be extended superiorly in certain patients. The goal will be to cross the non–hair-bearing expanse of skin from the posterior sulcus to the hairline at a position that the ear in the normal position will hide the scar. The scar then extends in the curvilinear fashion into the hairline. Typically this incision line corresponds to a line that would bisect the angle formed by a horizontal line from the superior external auditory canal and an inferior line of the hairline. A curvilinear incision then bisects the angle formed by this junction and nicely hides the incision within the hair-bearing skin itself. In very lax faces where more than 2 cm of skin will require excision, the hairline may be better preserved if the incision follows the postauricular hairline margin for much of its extent and is then carried into the finer hair above the junction of the hair with the neck skin. The incision should not be left where it could be visible at the base of the hairline or in a position toward the anterior neck skin.

An important step in the postauricular incision is to irregularize the scar at the superior extent as the

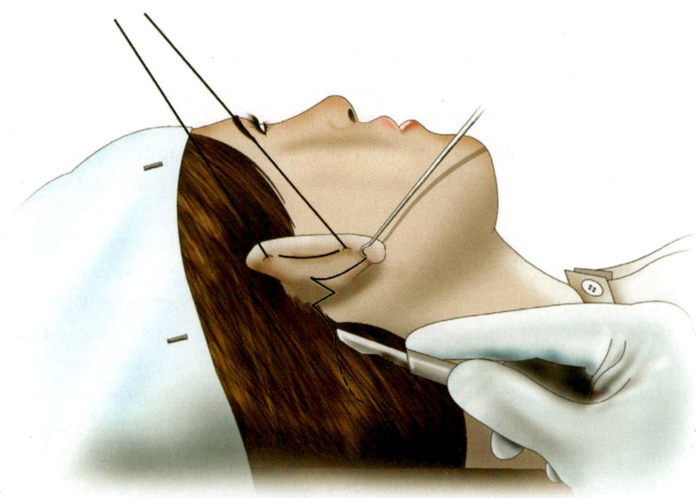

Figure 3-21. The postauricular incision is placed above the sulcus onto the concha and incorporates a small "V" as it crosses the sulcus superiorly.

incision crosses from the concha across postauricular sulci and to the occipital hairline. At this point, as noted, an irregularization in the form of a small V or a m-plasty is created. This maneuver both improves camouflage to the scar but importantly also avoids the possibility of a contracted bowstring scar or scar band across the same anatomic cavity.

Flap and SMAS Elevation

Following incision planning and facial marking, the area is injected with a local anesthetic. Infiltration of the anesthetic is completed on the side to be approached first. Typically 1% lidocaine with 1:100,000 epinephrine infiltrations are used. As noted earlier, surgery is typically performed under an intubated inhalation anesthesia and control of the airway during the procedure is seen as a safety precaution.

The amount of skin flap elevation must also be individualized for the patient's needs. Most patients benefit from what has been described as an "intermediate flap." This flap elevation is contrasted with a short flap, which may have just a few centimeters of undermining in the preauricular and subauricular area. It is also contrasted with a long flap, which may extend medially toward the midline of the face into or even beyond the nasolabial folds. The concept of the intermediate flap is that it allows good exposure to the superficial muscular aponeurotic system (SMAS) layer and redraping of the skin while at the same time avoids dissection in regions where the facial nerve branches will be more superficial and potentially of greater risk for injury. Similarly, this flap minimizes the amount of dead space remaining postoperatively and thus prevents the likelihood of hematoma. The degree and extent of flap elevation as described here is a key component of the Safety Facelift and has proven to minimize complication risk for the patient. The planned intermediate level of elevation thus is an area that begins beneath the approximate level of the zygomatic arch and extends out midway in the face approximately halfway between the auricle and the melolabial fold region (this is often approximately 6 cm in most patients). The same amount of undermining is extended inferiorly past the angle of the mandible into the neck from the inferior extent of the auricle and extends postauricularly into the occipital hair region. A good anatomic guideline is a landmark that corresponds to the level of the projection of the malar eminence. As noted previously, to extend undermining beyond this puts the facial nerve branches at risk as they become more superficial and accomplishes typically very little in terms of additional improvement of the facial appearance postoperatively.

Whether one begins flap development in the temporal and preauricular region or the postauricular elevation is largely surgeon preference. It has been found to be helpful to initially make the incision from the temporal preauricular, postauricular, and occipital regions and establish the incision and then return to begin to elevate flap in a regional approach. Most often the temporal region is elevated first. It is important that this be at a level inferior to the hair follicles. In this temporal aesthetic unit, elevation can proceed with relative ease and particularly in the primary patient with little or no bleeding under direct vision using blunt instrument elevation. The proper plane of elevation is deep to the hair follicles, which most readily is developed superficial to the temporal fascia and in the loose tissue plane over the fascia. Spreading with a blunt instrument such as a hemostat often accomplishes most of the elevation (**see Figures 3-22 and 3-23**).

An important note at this point is that the elevation in the temporal area need not go beyond the temporal hairline itself. Experience has shown that correction in the lateral orbital region and upper aspects of the facelift can be accomplished appropriately without further elevation. By limiting the elevation within the hairline, several important aspects of the Safety Facelift approach are accomplished. First, it helps to maintain temporal hairline and hair tuft position. Second, and importantly, it avoids the temporal branch of the facial nerve. The flap then carefully avoids significant elevation onto the zygomatic arch where, again, the facial nerve would be at risk. Below the zygomatic arch, the flap is elevated and the subcutaneous plane and extended to the intermediate position as described. With appropriate injection, bleeding is typically minimal in this area and any bleeding points encountered can be easily controlled with a pinpoint bipolar cautery. This facial cheek flap in the subcutaneous plane ensues with maintenance of a layer of fat preserved on the flap to preserve the subdermal vascular plexus and ensure uniform redraping of the elevated skin. Gentle flap retraction by the surgeon and the assistant using wide double tissue hooks minimizes the trauma associated with other types of retractors. Most of the elevation in the cheek flap area is accomplished by gentle scissor spreading,

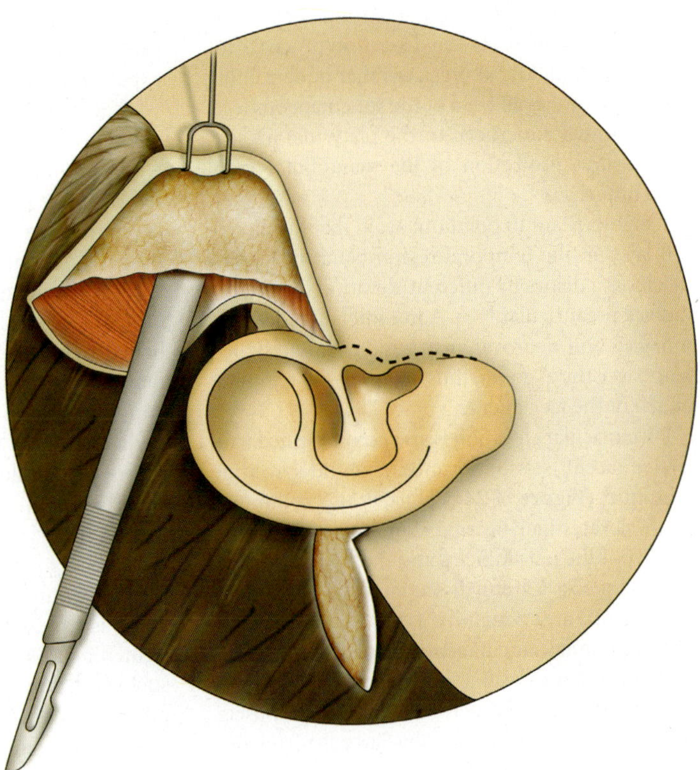

Figure 3-22. The temporal region flap elevation is deep to the hair follicles and above the superficial temporal fascia. It does not extend beyond the hairline.

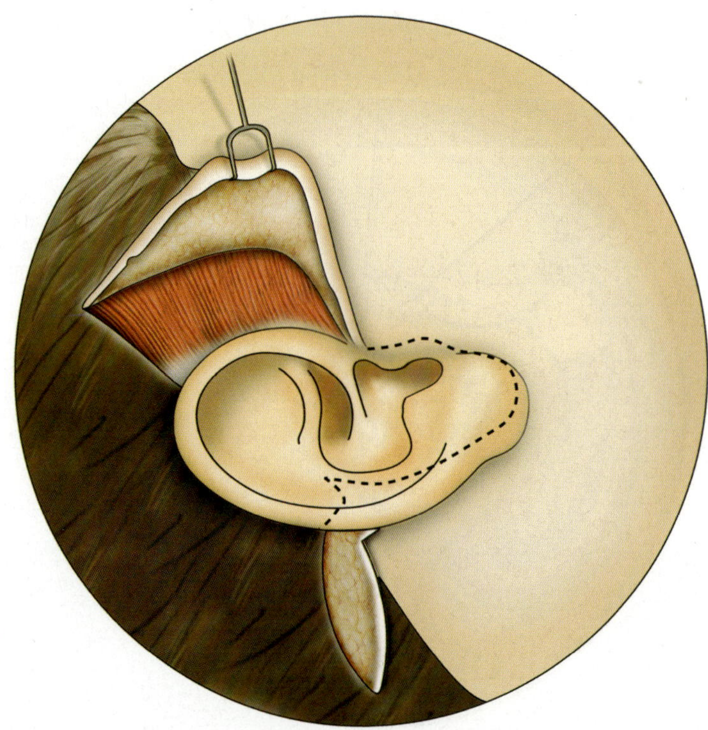

Figure 3-23. Flap retraction with wide double tissue hooks facilitate the elevation and minimizes flap skin trauma.

and very little actual division or cutting of the tissue is typically required. As the dissection proceeds inferiorly, it should be appreciated that undermining at this juncture as all been at the subcutaneous level and continues superficial to the platysmal muscle. This ensures protection of the mandibular facial nerve branch.

It is important to point out again that the dissection layer in the temporal region beneath the hair follicles is a distinctly different elevation than in the midface preauricular area. A noninterrupted bridge of SMAS and neurovascular bundle should be left intact over the zygoma, thus avoiding the temporal branch of the facial nerve.

Postauricular elevation is also accomplished with beveled facelift scissor advancement and spreading technique (**Figure 3-24**). During the technique, which elevates hair-bearing skin, one should carefully avoid the hair follicles and thus avoid postoperative alopecia. Careful dissection in the immediate postauricular area is required as this is a region where there is minimal subcutaneous tissue and the skin is both quite thin as well as adherent to the fascia as it extends down to the sternocleidomastoid muscle. Careful attention separating this layer is of key importance. Attention should be focused at this point to avoid branches of the greater auricular nerve. As the dissection, continues inferiorly, it is joined with the anterior dissection beneath the lobule of the ear. Following a precise hemostasis with bipolar cautery under direct vision, the SMAS layer is now exposed (**Figure 3-25**).

Elevation of the SMAS layer presents the surgeon with several alternatives. In the occasional patient with minimum laxity (typically in the younger patient) simple plication of the SMAS may be all that is required. In this situation 3-0 PDS sutures with buried knots are utilized to achieve elevation of the soft tissues and thus allow for redraping the redundant skin. Most facelift patients, however, will benefit more from incision and elevation of the SMAS tissue with subsequent repositioning, tightening, and imbrication with strong absorbable sutures such as 3-0 PDS. Some surgeons prefer a permanent suture for plication; however, with longer lasting absorbable sutures, wound strength is maintained until appropriate healing has occurred and the concern of later palpable sutures or even sutures "spitting" is eliminated. The SMAS layer is elevated only as far as required for appropriate repositioning and tightening. Further undermining beyond this area such as is done with various so-called deep-plane procedures does not seem to significantly add to postoperative results and puts facial nerve branches at risk (**Figures 3-26, 3-27, 3-28, and 3-29**).

Inferiorly, the SMAS becomes the confluent with the platysmal area and, in the same sub-SMAS platysmal plane, the inferior tissues are also elevated

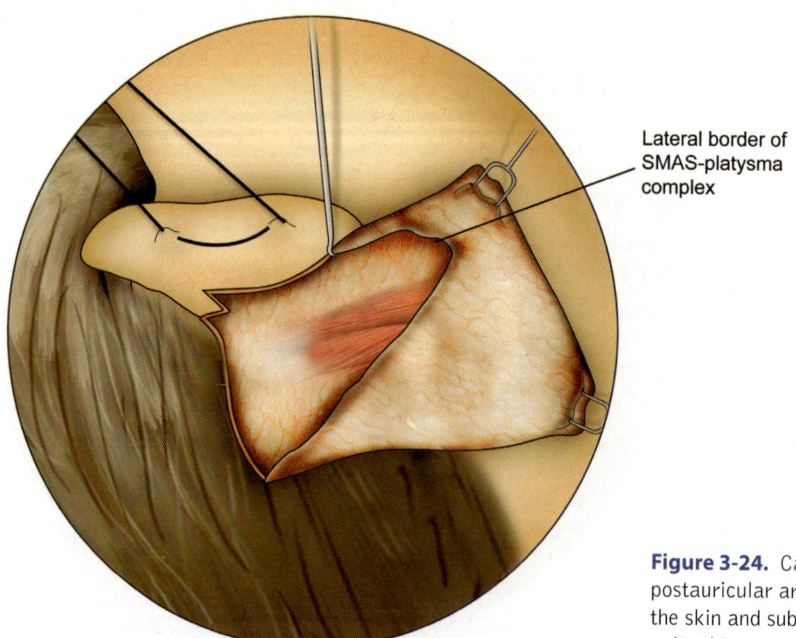

Figure 3-24. Careful dissection in the postauricular area is required where the skin and subcutaneous layer is quite thin.

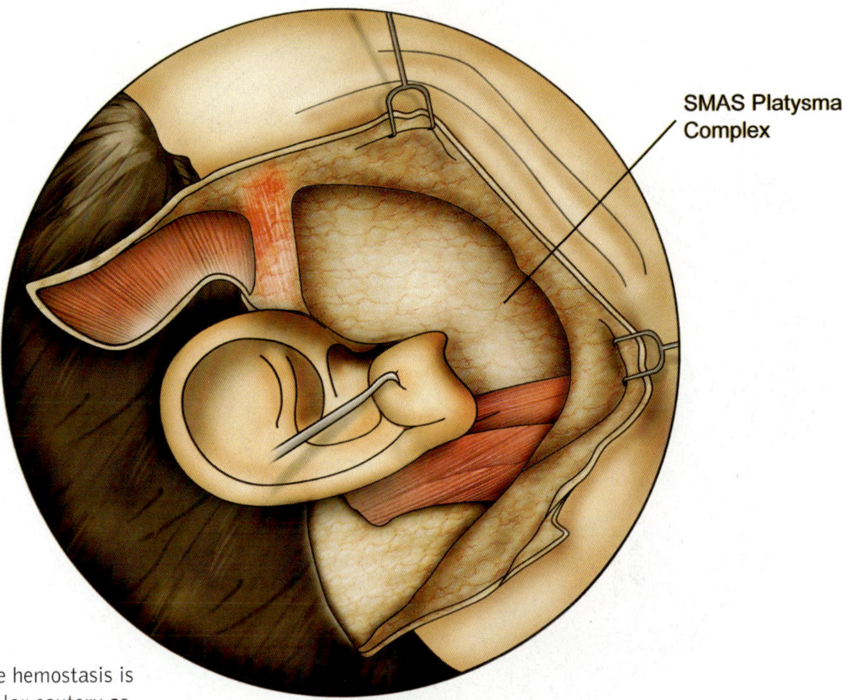

Figure 3-25. Precise hemostasis is maintained with bipolar cautery as the SMAS layer is exposed.

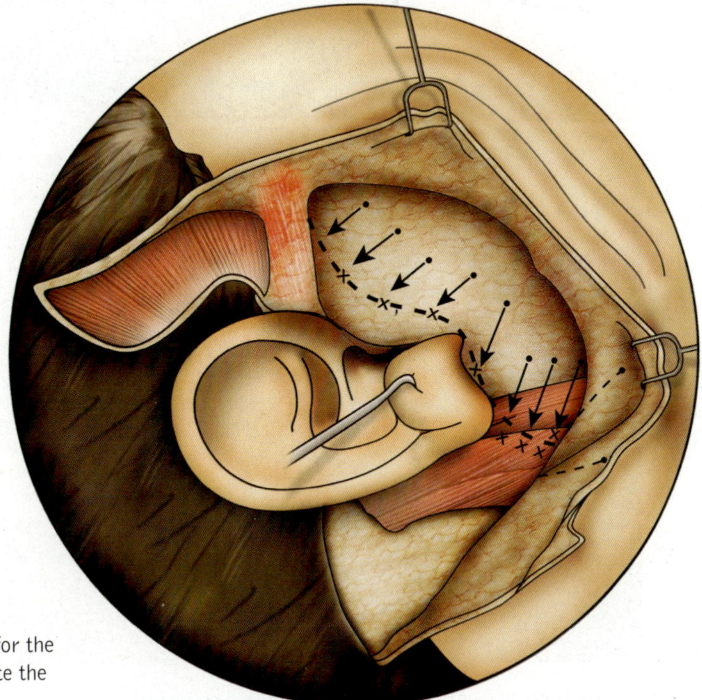

Figure 3-26. Typical incision line for the SMAS and platysmal complex. Note the two different vectors of the flap.

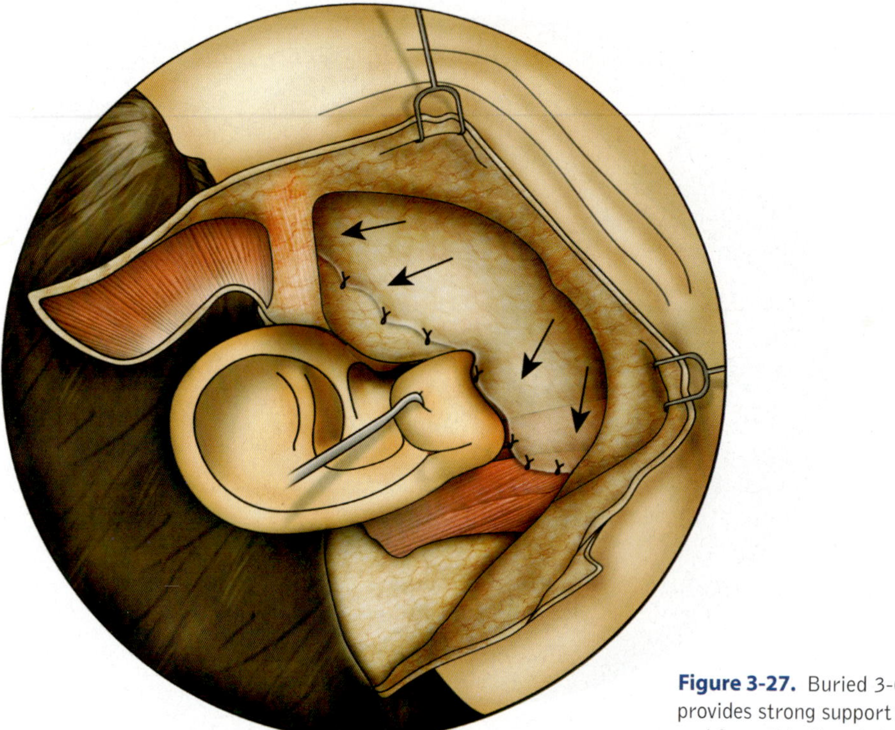

Figure 3-27. Buried 3-0 PDS suture provides strong support until healing and favorable fibrosis has occurred.

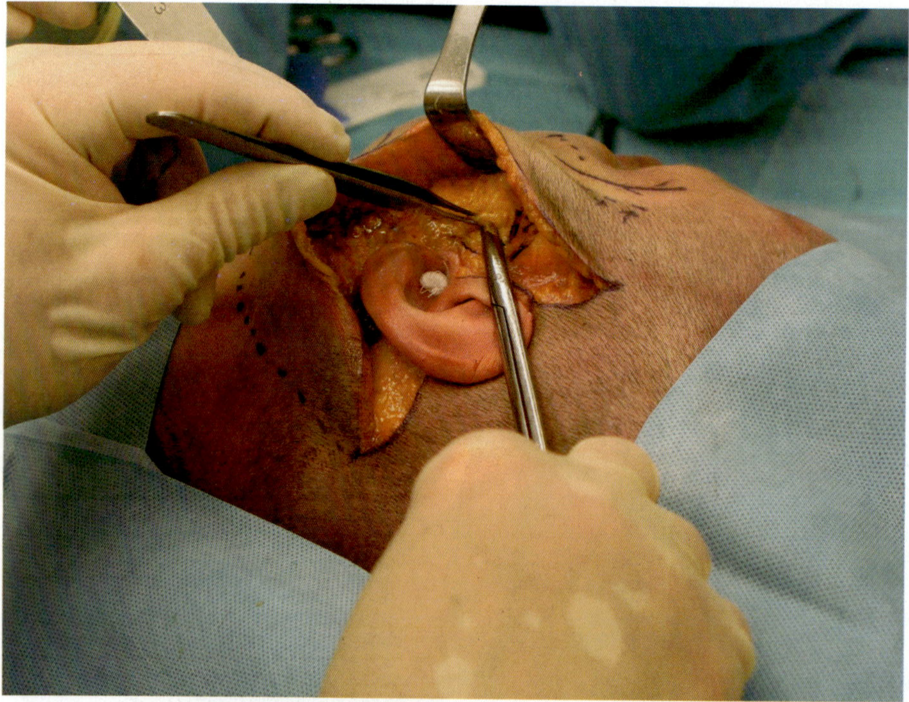

Figure 3-28. Facial flap elevation in a cadaver preparation reveals the SMAS layer.

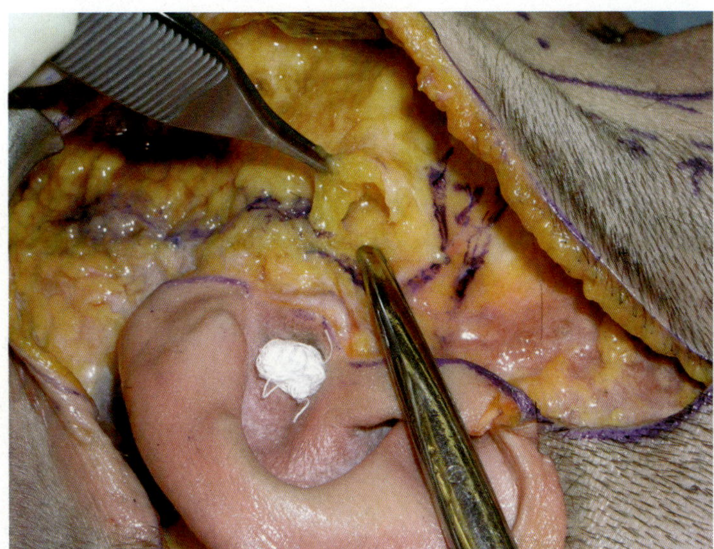

Figure 3-29. The SMAS layer undermining is initiated inferior to the zygomatic arch.

for tightening of the mandibular and submandibular neck region. The amount of undermining required to appropriately tighten and reposition facial features is periodically checked with strong retraction. Once that level has been obtained, this area of tissue can be excised in preparation for imbrication. When an appropriate level of this conservative elevation of the midface tissues has been completed, direct vision of the movement of the facial tissues is then used. At this point the "two-vector" approach provides best results in that the midface area will require a different direction and rector of pull than the postauricular and lower facial SMAS layer. Often, in patients with significant redundant tissue, the SMAS flap is divided at the level of the inferior auricular attachment so that there is a superior midface component and an inferior postauricular neck component. These patients frequently require different vectors of support, suspension, and correction.

With an assistant holding the elevated flap in position, redundant SMAS tissue is excised and key sutures are placed to hold the SMAS platysmal complex layer in the proper position using interrupted 3-0 PDS sutures with the knots buried. Once the entire redundant amount of SMAS has been excised and key sutures are placed, these sutures are then reinforced with additional sutures. In effect, now the redundant SMAS has been trimmed and the excess removed and the remaining SMAS flap sutured edge to edge with absorbable monofilament suture material. This maneuver has additional advantage when combined with the intermediate skin flap elevation to begin to eliminate significant amounts of dead space. Because the skin flap has not been elevated beyond that area, there is minimal potential for bleeding to occur or hematoma to accumulate. At this stage, the patient will be noted to have had a significant lifting and tightening force on facial and cervical skin and significant improvement in appearance even before skin excision has been accomplished.

Excision and Closure

After elevation, excision, and closure of the SMAS facial layer, the skin flap can now be redraped and excess redundant skin excised. Again, multiple vectors are required for best redraping of the skin and typically a two-vector approach is used. The temporal and preauricular skin is advanced and closed with a different vector of tension than the infra-auricular and postauricular skin flap. In order to avoid a pulled or artificial look, it is important that the skin essentially be redraped with minimal tension. The advantage of the tight two-vector SMAS lift is that it allows the skin to be repositioned, elevated, and redraped without tension on the skin itself. This also has the advantage of creating minimal tension on wound closure, thus resulting in better scars as well as avoiding the so-called stretched or windblown look postoperatively (**Figures 3-30, 3-31, and 3-32**).

Once the suture repositioning of the SMAS layer has created a satisfactory effect with good support,

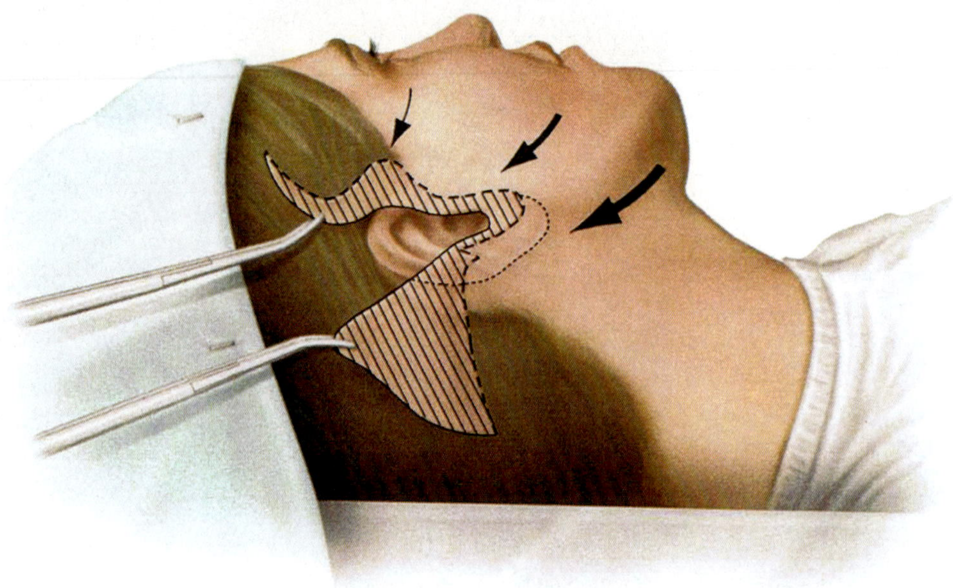

Figure 3-30. The skin is redraped with minimal tension in a two-vector directional fashion.

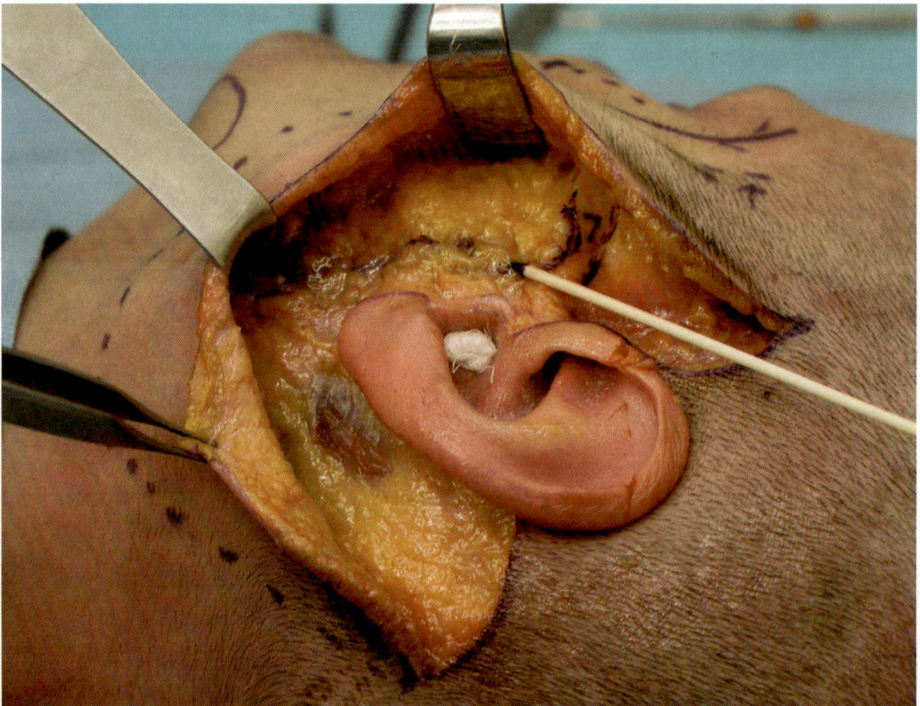

Figure 3-31. Incision line in the SMAS layer is indicated in blue and extends into the posterior platysmal margin.

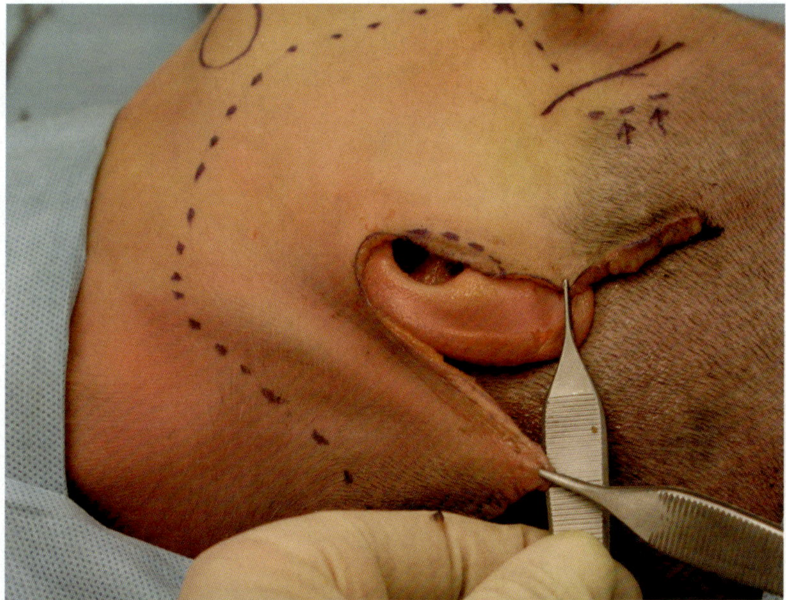

Figure 3-32. Redundant excess skin is excised.

the skin flaps are then placed on light traction and the vector forces the skin flap repositioning are assessed. It is important to avoid significant repositioning of the side burn or temporal hair area. Skin is then repositioned under minimal or no tension and two key sutures are put into place. The first key suture is at the superior helix attachment area at the temporal region and the second at the junction of the scalp hairline in the non–hair-bearing expanse of postauricular skin (**Figures 3-33 and 3-34**). Once these sutures are in place, there is no further tension required on the skin flap and it can

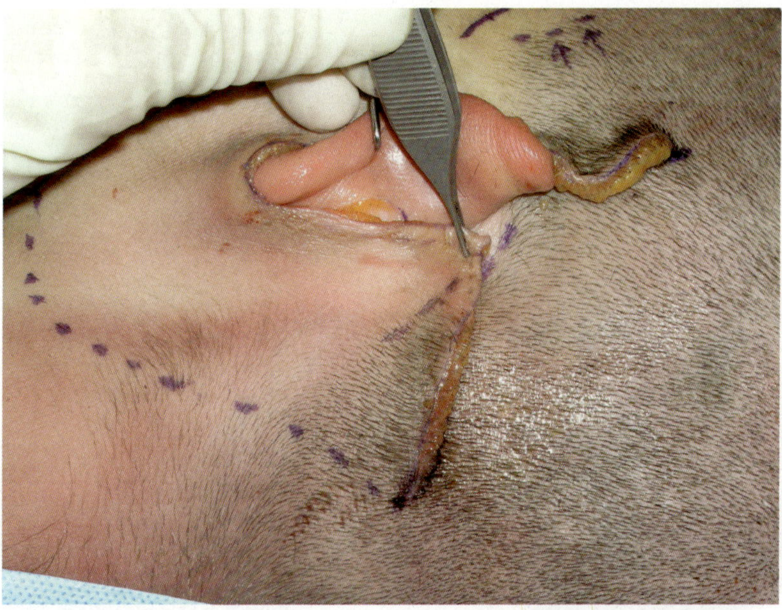

Figure 3-33. The Postauricular flap is carefully positioned to align the hairline.

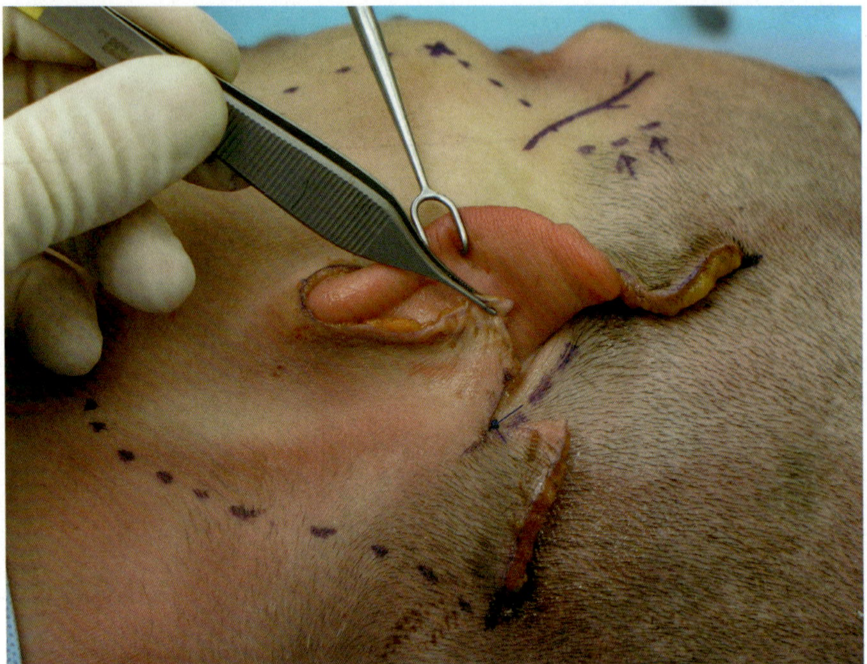

Figure 3-34. A key suture is placed at the hairline to maintain flap position.

be precisely tailored away for edge-to-edge positioning without tension on the wound closure (**Figure 3-35**). At this point, it is clear that the facelift elevation is being accomplished through the SMAS layer and does not depend on the facial skin for tightening. It is critical in the postauricular area to position the skin so it avoids a stepoff at the postauricular hairline. Following placement of the key sutures, the skin along the postauricular occipital region is incised in a beveled fashion to preserve

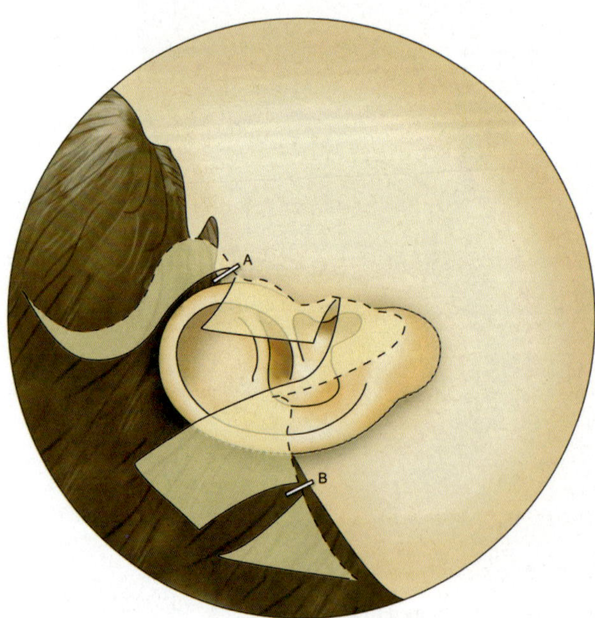

Figure 3-35. Key sutures are placed to position the skin flap with minimal tension.

hair follicles, and this incision is usually closed in a single layer using small surgical staples. The skin in the non–hair-bearing postauricular region is sutured with a running 5-0 fast-absorbing gut suture. The temporal hair-bearing area has skin excised in similar fashion and again closed with small skin staples. The earlobe is positioned so that there is a sense of tucking flap underneath the earlobe and without tension in that region to avoid distortion of the lobe or a visible scar. The preauricular tissue is again excised in an edge-to-edge fashion without tension and the tragal flap is developed. The skin over the tragus is thinned down to the subdermal plexus to allow for appropriate conforming of soft tissue to the tragus to avoid a thicker postoperative look. A single layer of closure is all that is required here because of the lack of tension. The superior and inferior preauricular incision is closed with a running 5-0 Prolene suture in the subcuticular layer. The posttragal incision after careful trimming and tailoring is closed with a running locked 6-0 fast-absorbing gut suture. The final step of tailoring is done along the postauricular sulcus where, following excision of the excess skin, it is closed with a running locked 5-0 fast-absorbing suture. This creates minimal response in the skin and allows the patient and surgeon to avoid suture removal on these sites. Because of the relatively small amount of undermined space following tight SMAS correction and modest flap elevation, usually no drain is required (**Figure 3-36**). Precise hemostasis with bipolar cautery throughout the procedure is essential as an additional component to avoid this drain requirement (**Figures 3-37–3-43**).

Postoperative Dressing

Upon completion of the surgical procedure, the wound margins are meticulously cleaned and antibiotic ointment applied to the areas. Elastics that have held the hair in proper position are removed and the hair is washed and rinsed as required. A fluff dressing is placed over the facial areas including postauricular and submental regions and then an elastic gauze dressing is applied followed by a minimally constrictive elastic wrap. The circumferential dressing goes beneath the chin and over the occipital area of the head. Care is taken to make sure the dressing is firm but not overly constrictive.

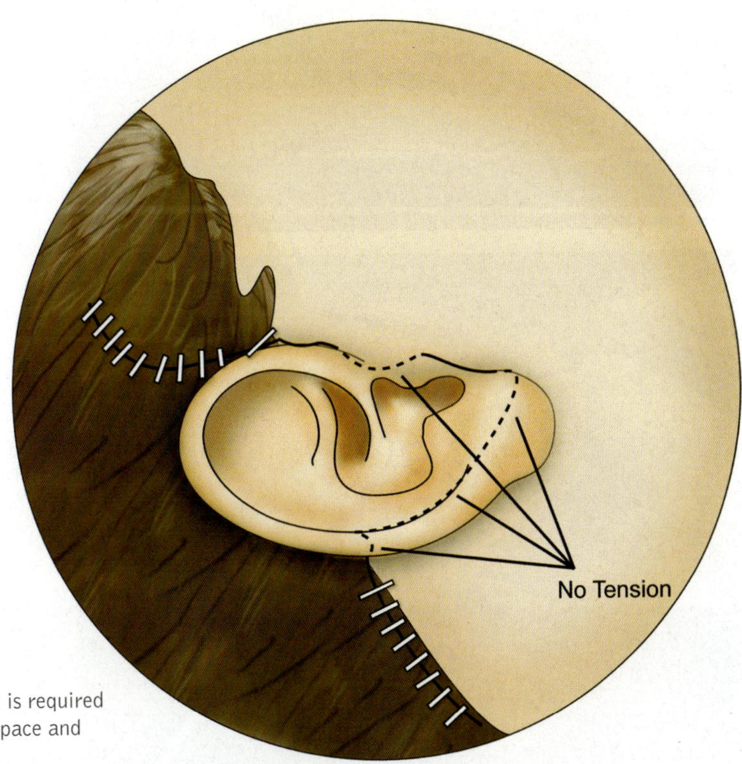

Figure 3-36. Typically no drain is required due to the modest undermined space and precise hemostasis.

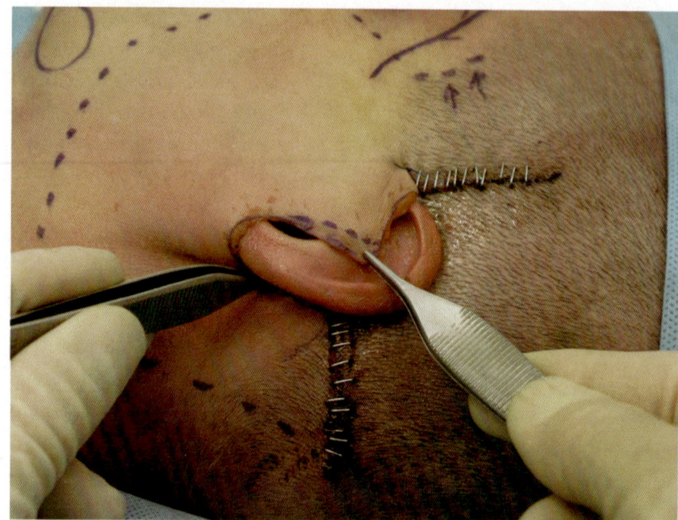

Figure 3-37. Following excision and closure of the temporal and postauricular flaps, the amount of preauricular skin to be excised is determined.

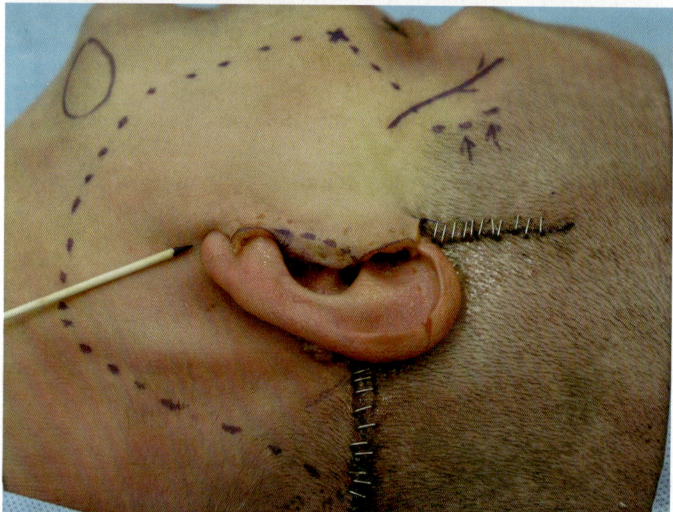

Figure 3-38. Earlobe is positioned so that the flap is tucked beneath the lobule and closed without tension.

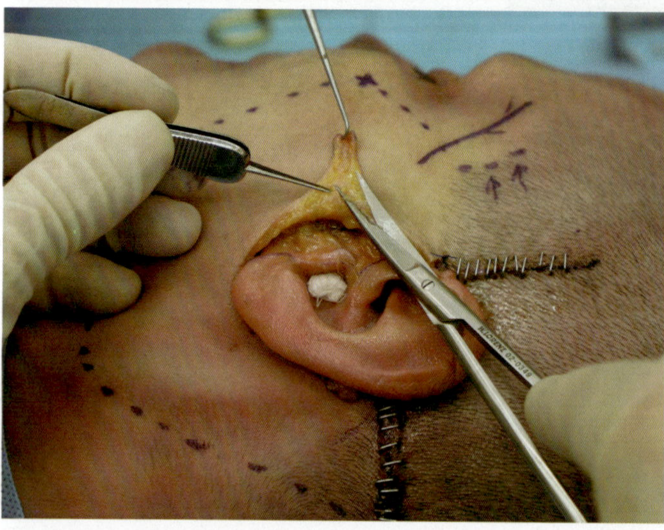

Figure 3-39. Tragal flap is thinned to avoid and overly thickened appearance.

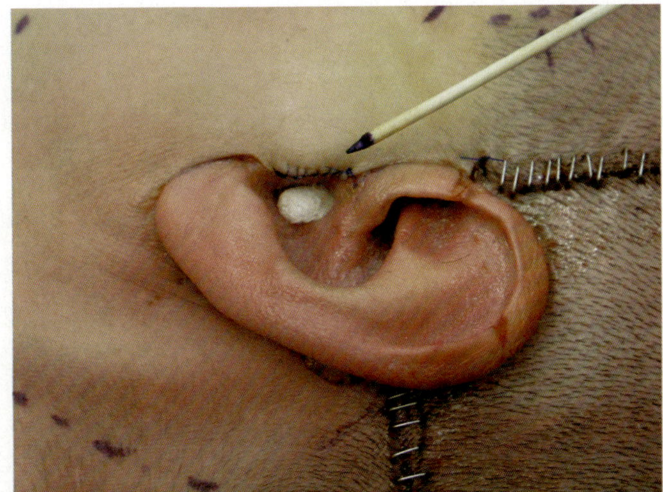

Figure 3-40. The posttragal closure is accomplished with absorbable 6-0 suture in running locked fashion (shown in blue for demonstration).

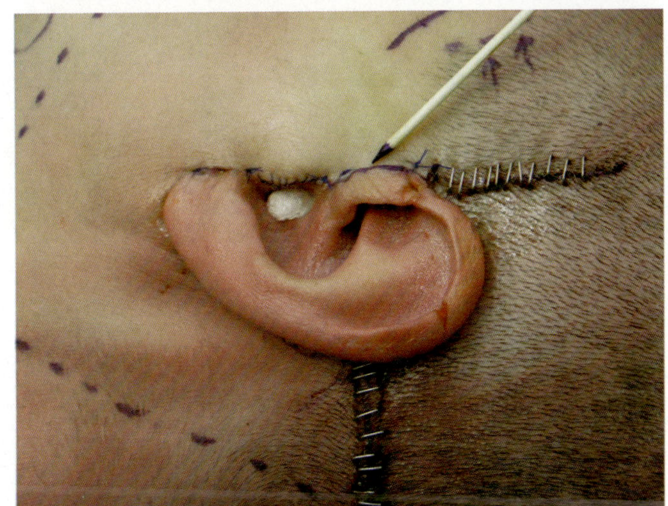

Figure 3-41. The superior and inferior portion of the incision is closed with a single layer in a running intracuticular 5-0 suture.

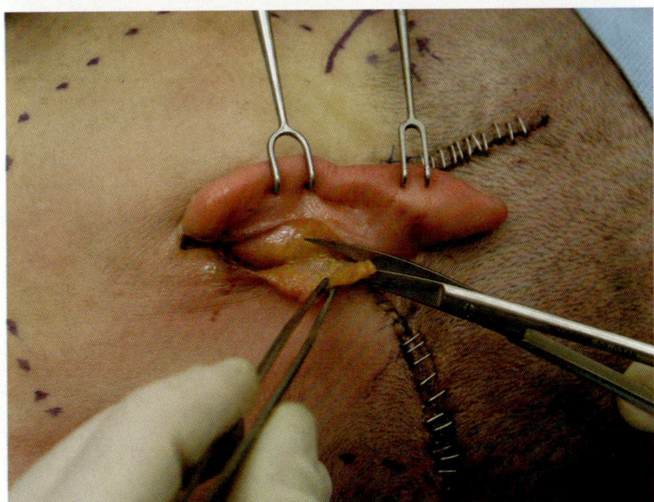

Figure 3-42. The superior and inferior portion of the incision is closed with a single layer in a running intracuticular 5-0 suture.

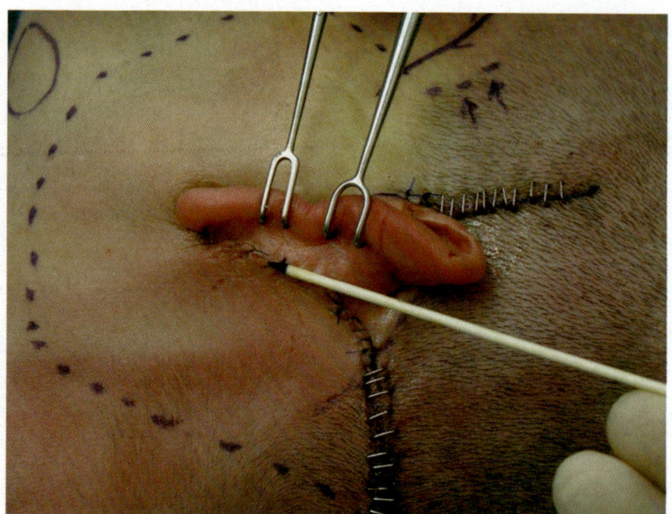

Figure 3-43. Postauricular closure is done with a running absorbable 5-0 suture.

References

1. Ehlert TK, Thomas JR, Becker FF. Submental W-plasty for correction of turkey gobbler deformities. *Arch Otolaryngol.* 1990, 116, 714–717.
2. Thomas JR. Facial plastic surgery applications for liposuction, in Cummings, et al (eds.), *Otolaryngology: Head and Neck Surgery*. 3rd ed. St. Louis, Mosby-Yearbook 1990, 160–165.
3. Kridel RW, Liv ES. Techniques for creative inconspicuous facelift scars. *Arch Facial Plast Surg.* 2003, 5, 325–333.

4

Postoperative Care

In the immediate postoperative period and for 24 hours after, the patient is asked to keep the head elevated. Nonaspirin-containing analgesics are provided along with an antibiotic and antinausea medication as required. Patients are checked the evening of surgery and the morning following surgery, the dressing is removed, and the patient is inspected for a hematoma. A circumferential dressing is reapplied for an additional 24 hours and if the patient shows no sign of hematoma or other difficulties, the dressing is removed on the second postoperative day. The patient is given an elastic chin support that can be removed for bathing but otherwise retained for the remainder of one week.

Incisions are kept covered with antibiotic ointment, which is applied twice a day for 1 week; oral antibiotics (cephalosporin 500 mg twice daily) are provided for one week.

Gentle shampooing of the hair is allowed at 48–72 hours after surgery. Physical activities including lifting and active exercise are avoided for one week and then reinstituted gradually. Suture and staple removal is at 1 week. Absorbable sutures in the posttragal and postauricular regions dissolve over the 7–10 day postoperative period.

Patients are asked to minimize their activities during the first week. They are to keep their head elevated, use only warm water bathing and shampooing and avoid any strenuous activity including heavy lifting. The second week patients are allowed to return to normal bathing activities. They can return to normal skin care and return to physical exercise being careful primarily to avoid direct trauma to the facial skin. By week 2 the patients are allowed to return to all normal exercise and activity. They are asked to avoid hair coloring or other harsh hair chemicals for approximately 4 weeks. Finally, patients are warned to avoid sun exposure or other UV exposure for at least 3 months (**Figures 4-1 to 4-18**).

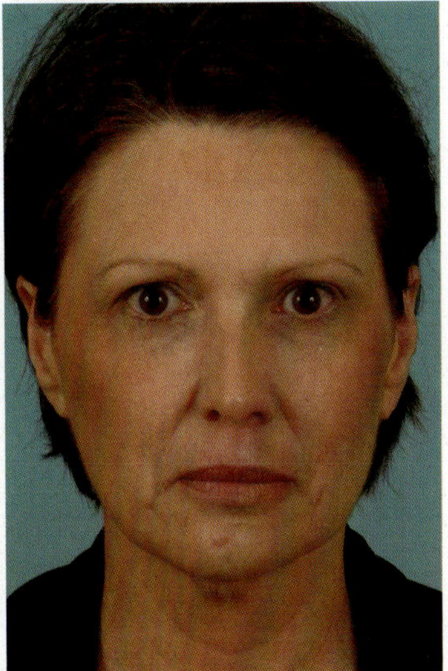

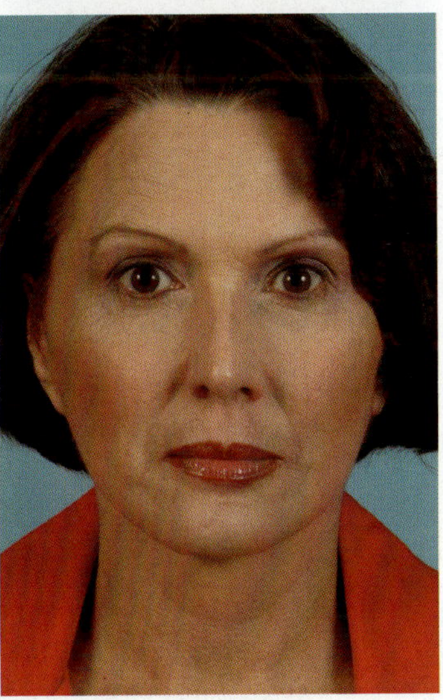

Figure 4-1 Pre- and postoperative views showing a more youthful but natural appearance achieved through the Safety Facelift.

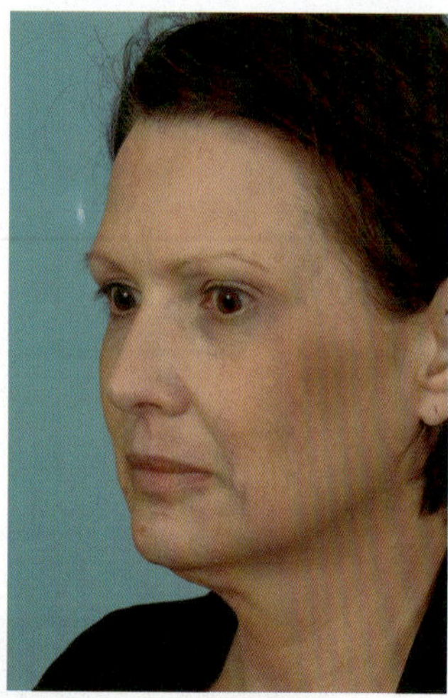

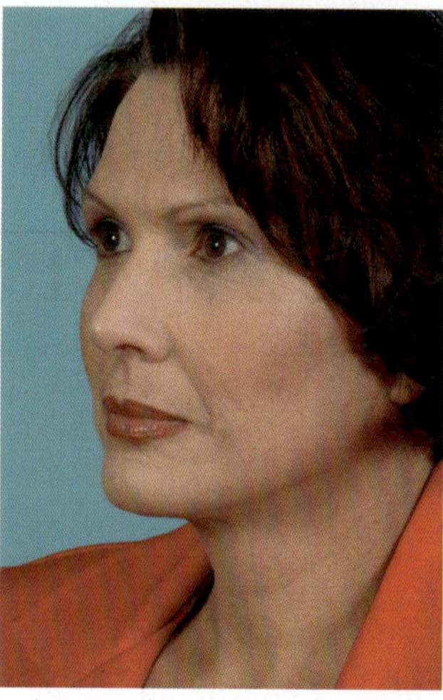

Figure 4-2 Improved midface, mandibular line, and submental regions while maintaining a natural appearance.

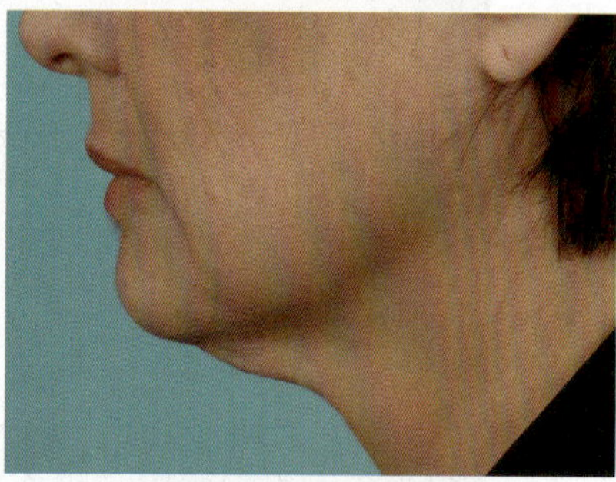

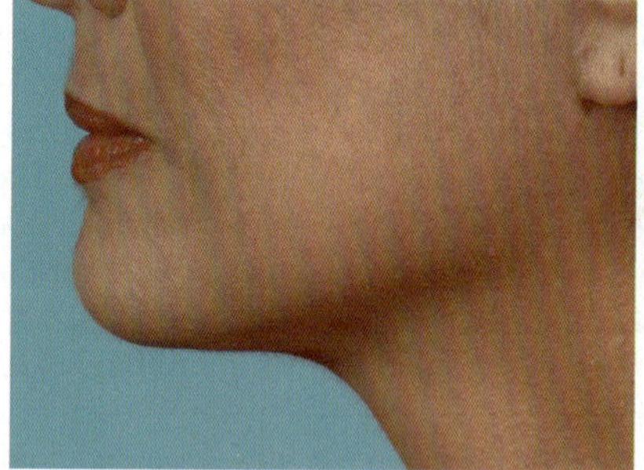

Figure 4-3 Close inspection of the lateral view reveals midface improvement combined with improved jawline appearance.

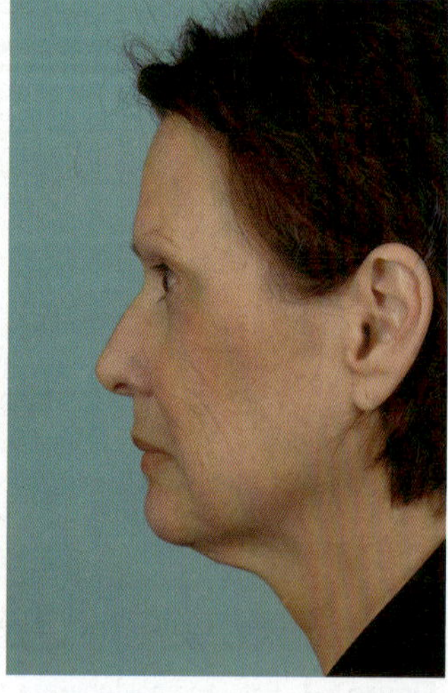

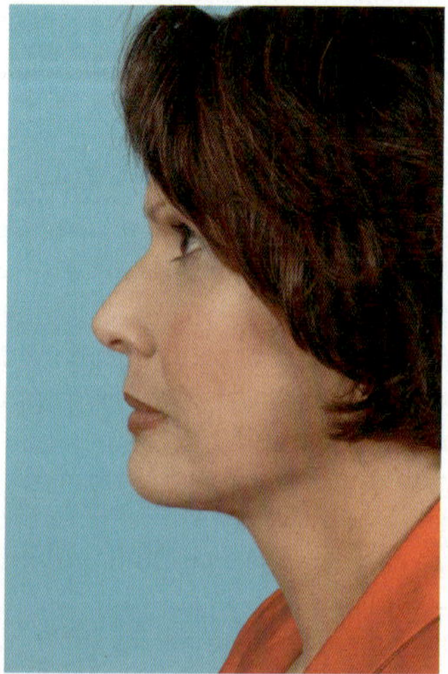

Figure 4-4 Lateral view displaying a natural improvement which is non-surgical in appearance in a typical patient.

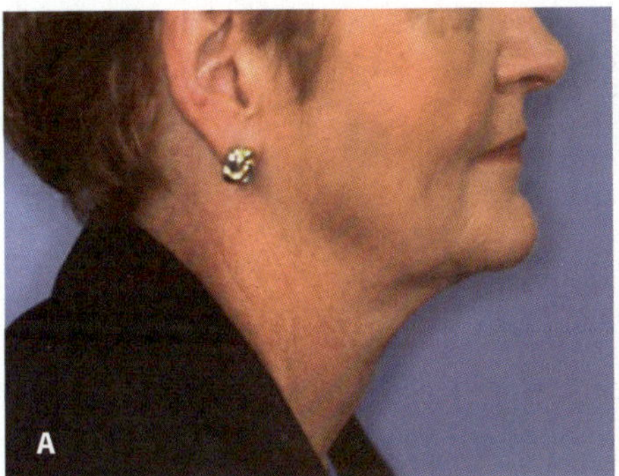

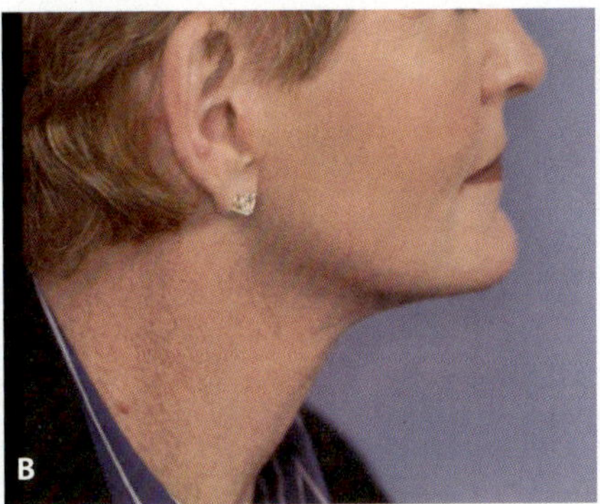

Figure 4-5 Preoperative loss of submental and mandibular elasticity (A), with postoperative improvements (B).

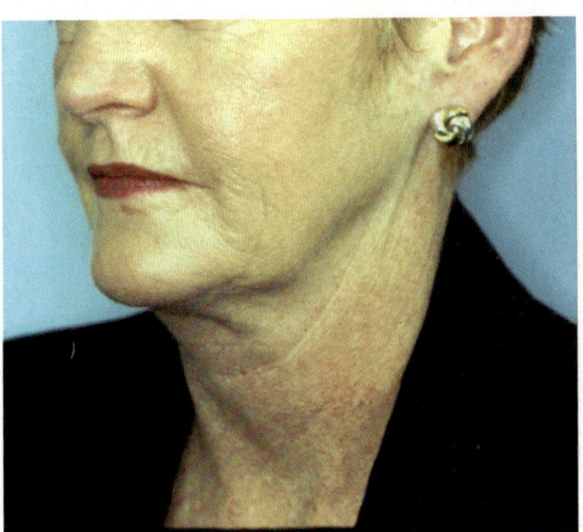

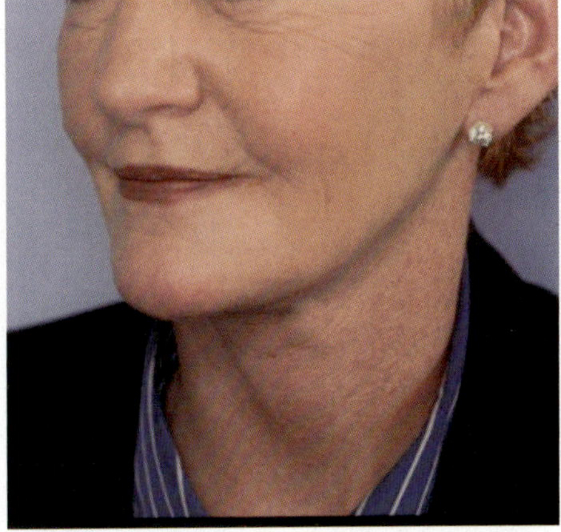

Figure 4-6 Postoperative view reveals natural improvement with well camouflaged incision.

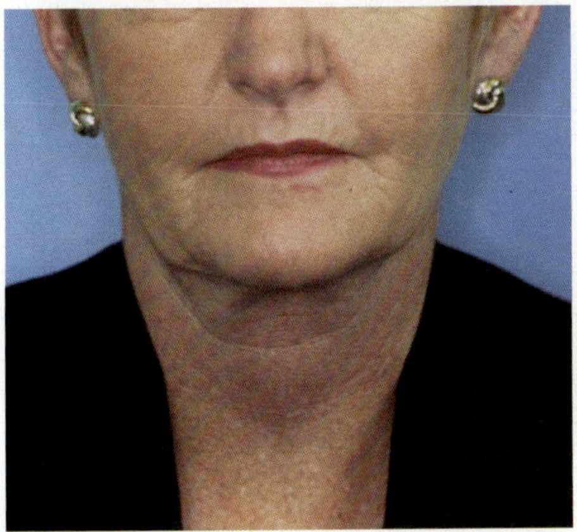

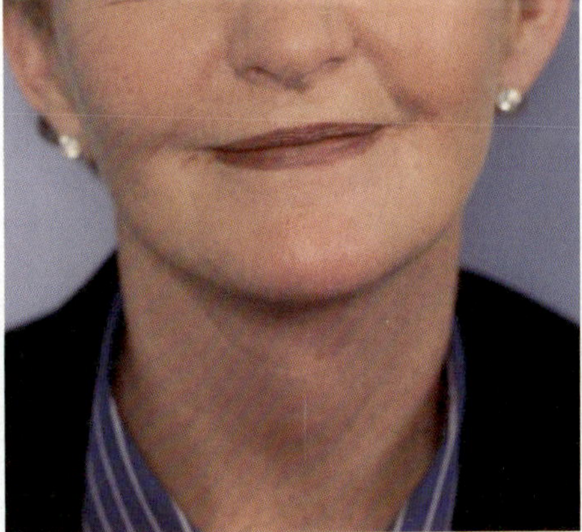

Figure 4-7 Improvement of platysmal bands and midface laxity.

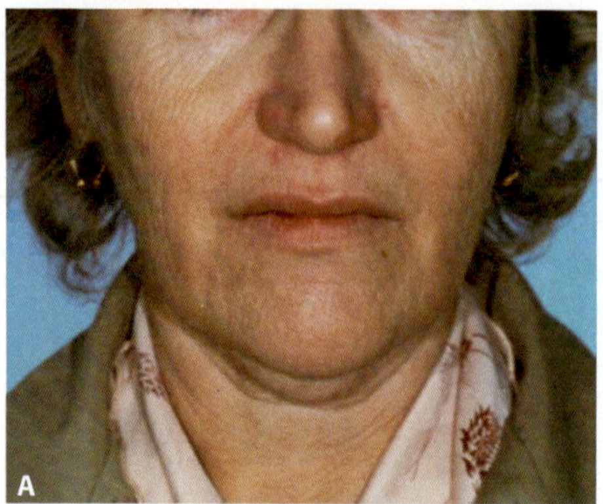

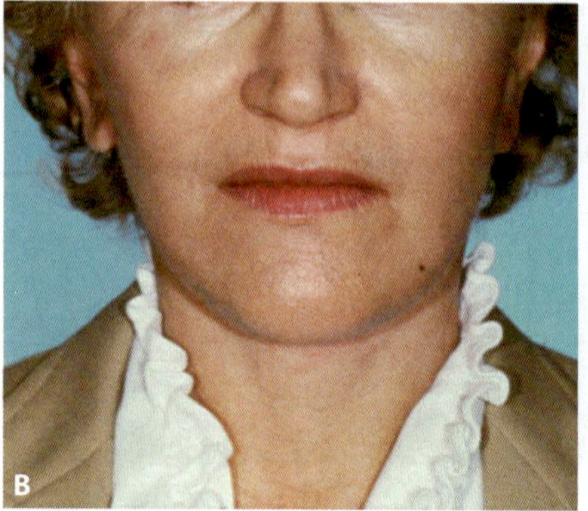

Figure 4-8 Significant submental laxity (A). Postoperative natural appearance improvement (B).

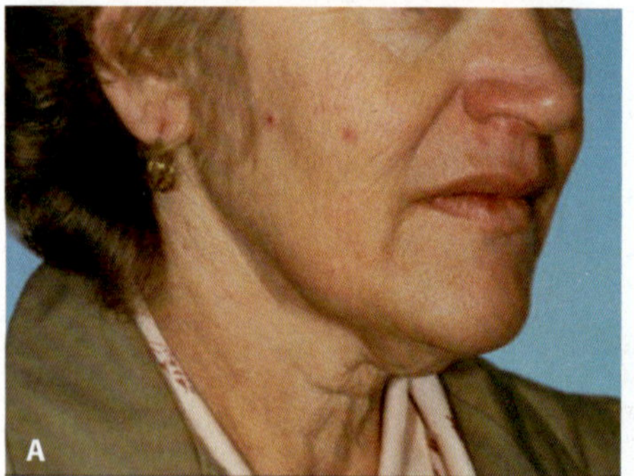

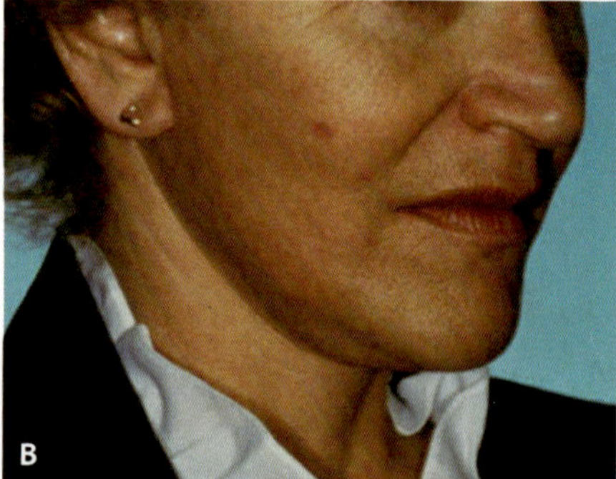

Figure 4-9 Mandibular line and submental areas improved (A) compared to pre op (B).

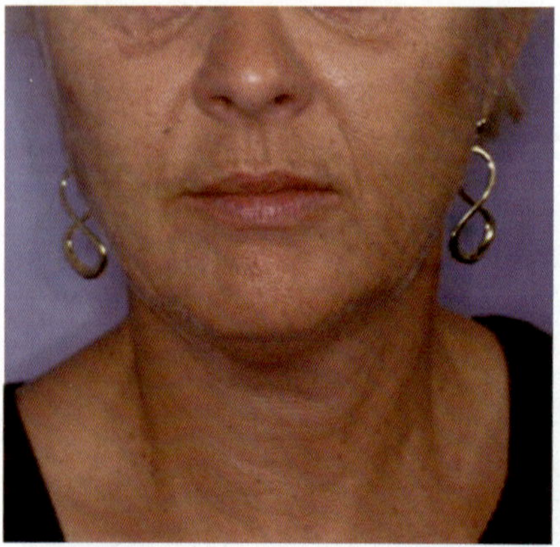

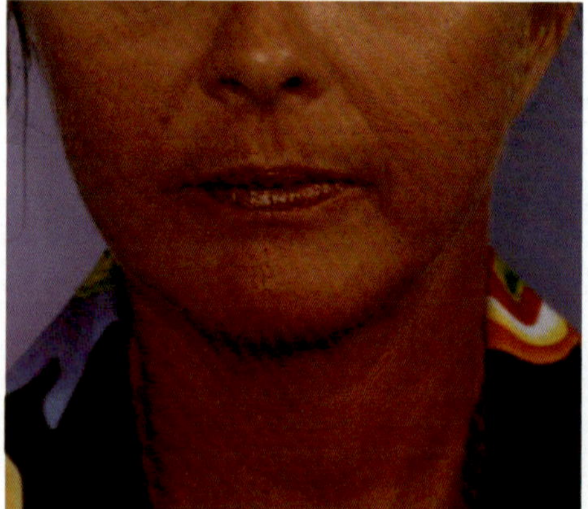

Figure 4-10 Pre- and postoperative views in patient with medium thickness skin.

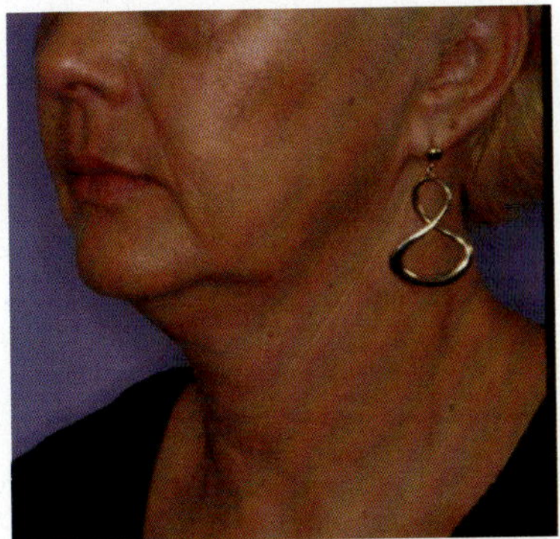
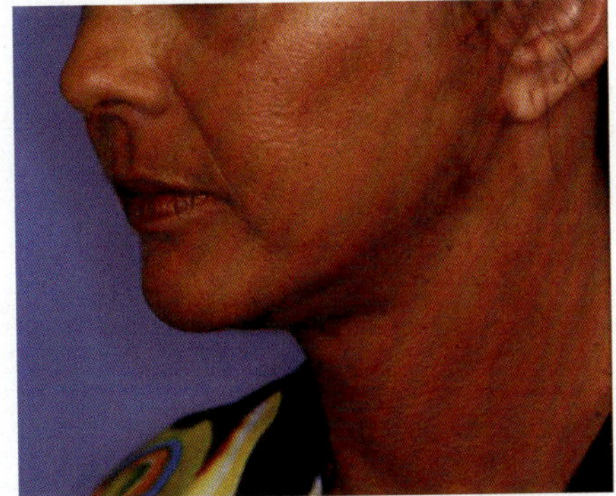

Figure 4-11 Creation of youthful cervicomental angle.

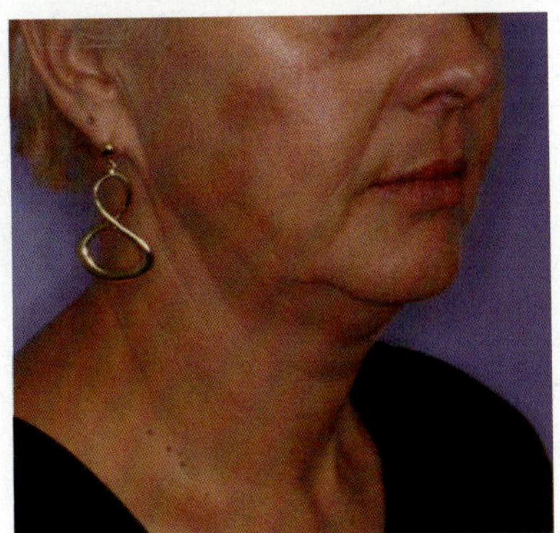
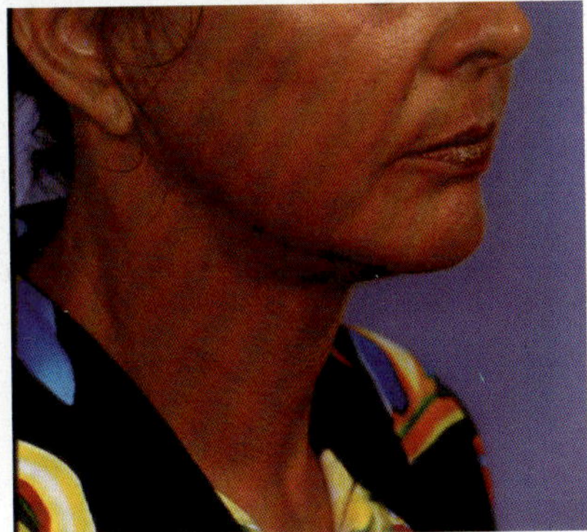

Figure 4-12 An improved jawline.

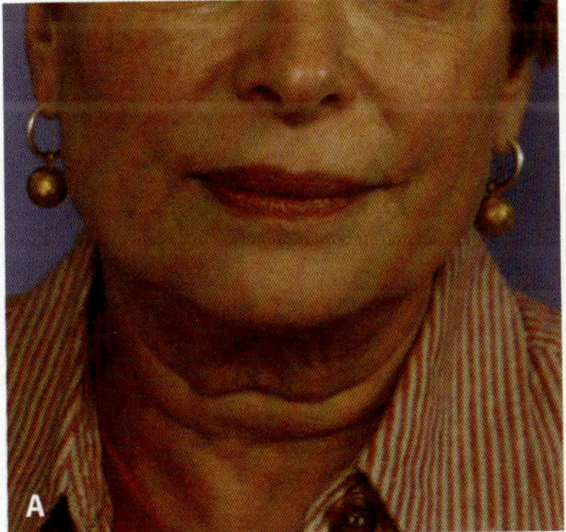
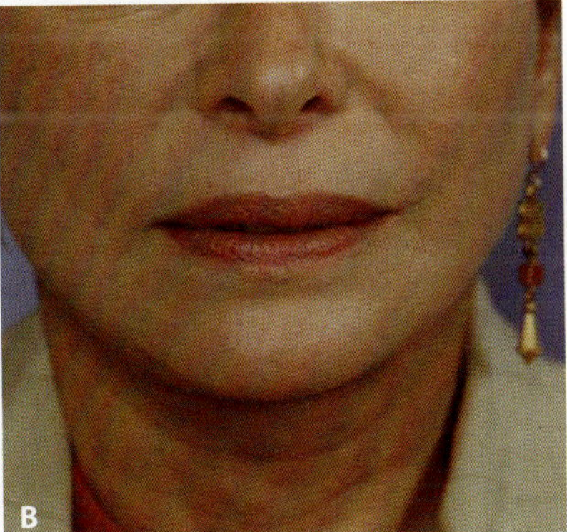

Figure 4-13 Preoperative soft tissue laxity of neck and submental region (A); postoperative improvements including neck skin (B).

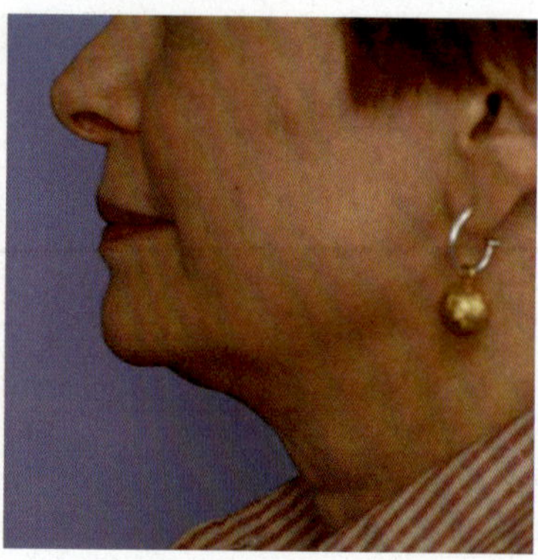

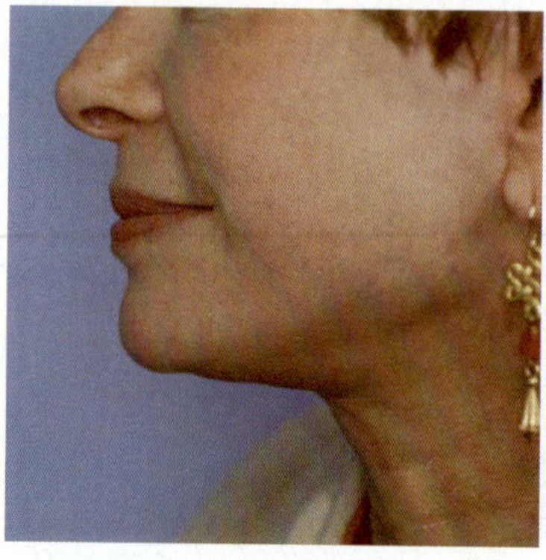

Figure 4-14 Creation of a youthful cervicomental angle post operatively.

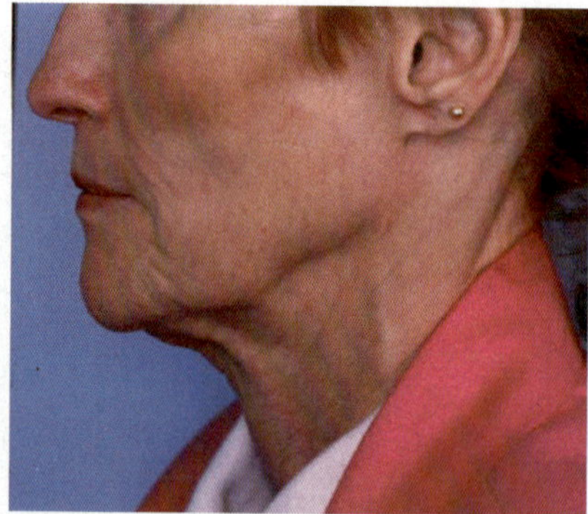

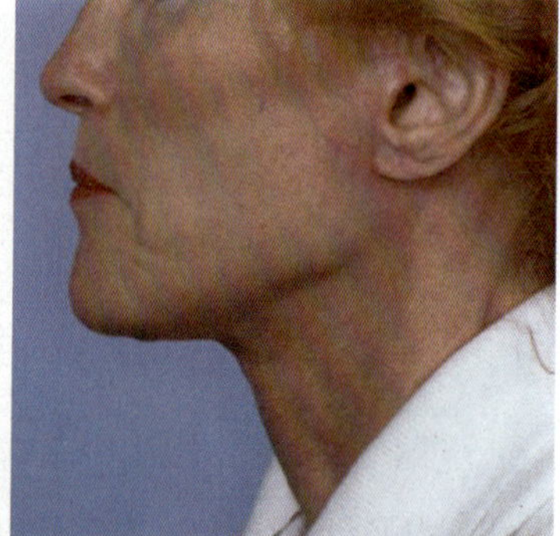

Figure 4-15 Patient with thin skin characteristics avoiding a "pulled" or "stretched" look post operatively.

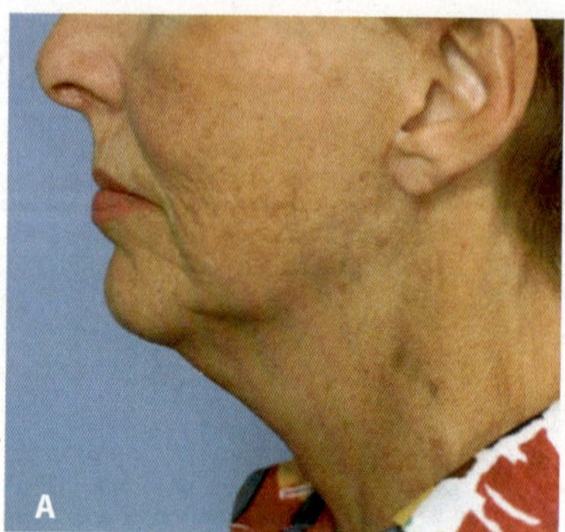

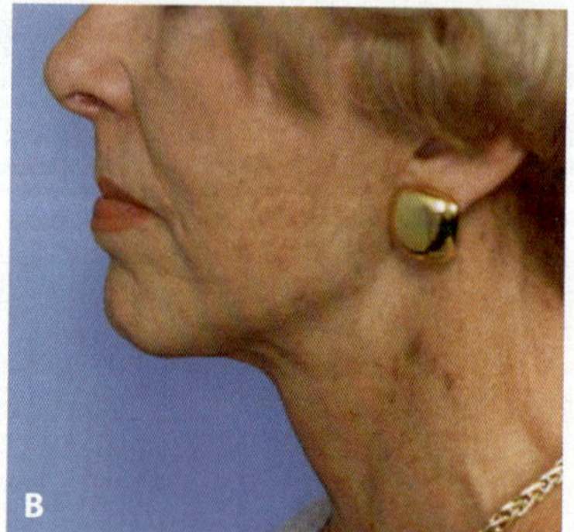

Figure 4-16 Preoperative (A) maintenance of cervicomental angle and mandibular line (B) several years post operatively.

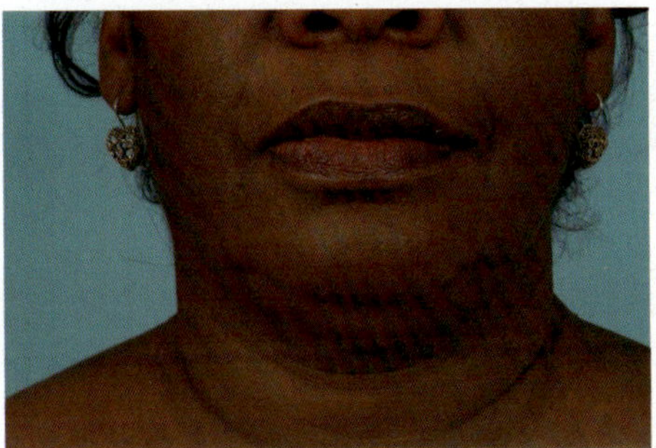
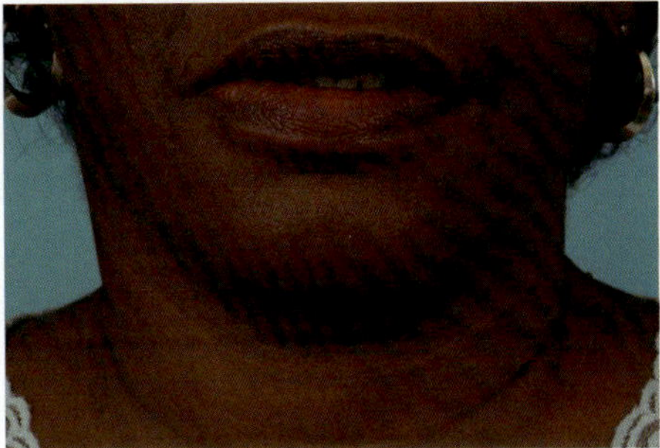

Figure 4-17 Postoperative improvement in a mildly obese patient with thick skin.

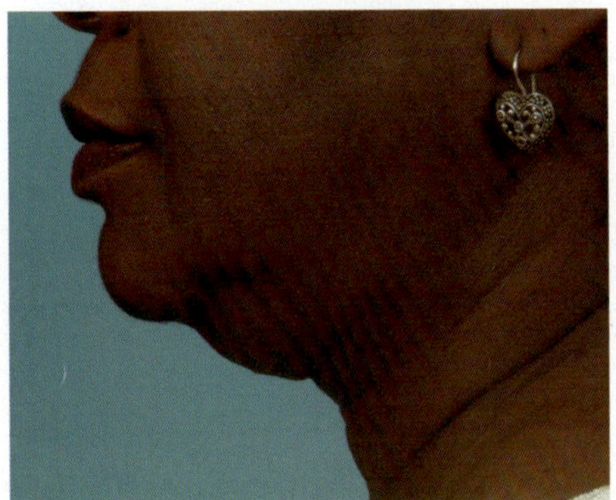
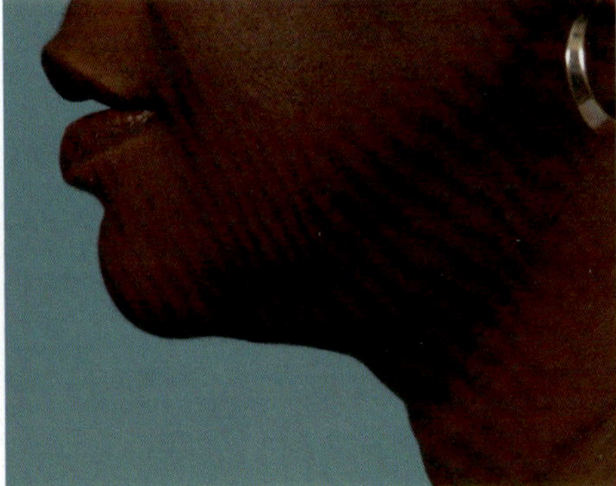

Figure 4-18 An improved chin and neck line in a thick-skinned patient.

5

COMPLICATIONS

Significant complications of facelift surgery are, fortunately, infrequent. Using the Safety Facelift concept as described in this book can help further minimize the complication rate. Steps used and discussed here are based on looking at various alternative procedures for facelifts and specific steps in the facelift procedure. For each of those steps, comparisons of various alternatives are evaluated and the alternative used, which gives an acceptable result with a minimum of risk. Assuming appropriate patient selection is done, including avoiding patients with bleeding disorders or systemic problems such as diabetes, the risk becomes less. External factors including smoking, use of aspirin or NSAID medications should also be avoided in the potential patient. Patients who smoke are told they need to be smoke free for a minimum of 3 months before surgery and to continue that for 3 months postoperatively.

The following are complications that should be the focus of the surgeon as well as discussed with the patient preoperatively.[1,2]

Hematoma

Hematoma is reportably the most common complication following a facelift and is reported to occur in 2–15% of patients according to the literature.[3] Using the Safety Facelift criteria along with proper patient selection as noted, hematoma has proven to be exceedingly unusual. An expanding hematoma in the first several hours following a facelift is a true surgical emergency. Prompt recognition and treatment significantly diminishes any possibility of poor healing as a result of the hematoma. A major hematoma requires reoperation and exploration on an emergency basis. Most hematomas occur in the first 6 or 8 hours following a facelift. In addition to inspection of the patient during that time frame, other hallmark signs that may indicate hematoma formation may include pain, nausea, swelling, and blood pressure elevation. Bleeding at the wound edge around the dressing is not necessarily a reliable indicator. Significant onset of pain should indicate a hematoma, particularly if it is associated with progressive swelling until proved otherwise. Ecchymoses, or bluish discoloration of the lips and lateral buccal mucosa, may also be physical signs of hematoma and should prompt closer inspection (**Figure 5-1**).

Delay in treatment of hematoma may lead to poor wound healing or even flap necrosis. Fluid accumulation from hematoma or seroma potentially leads to increase opportunity for infection. Treatment includes reexploration of the facial flap and treatment of any specific bleeding points. Often no specific bleeding area is identified and diffused oozing is found. Treatment consists of exploration, irrigation and clot evacuation, and cautery of any bleeding areas. Suction drain and a light pressure dressing should be reapplied.

More frequently, small or localized hematomas may be encountered that can be treated without returning to surgery. Simple aspiration and removal of the fluid with a 16-gauge needle under sterile conditions is often all that is required. Continuation of moderate pressure over the area is usually helpful. In these patients often an extended course of the antibiotic is prescribed and continued close inspection is in order.

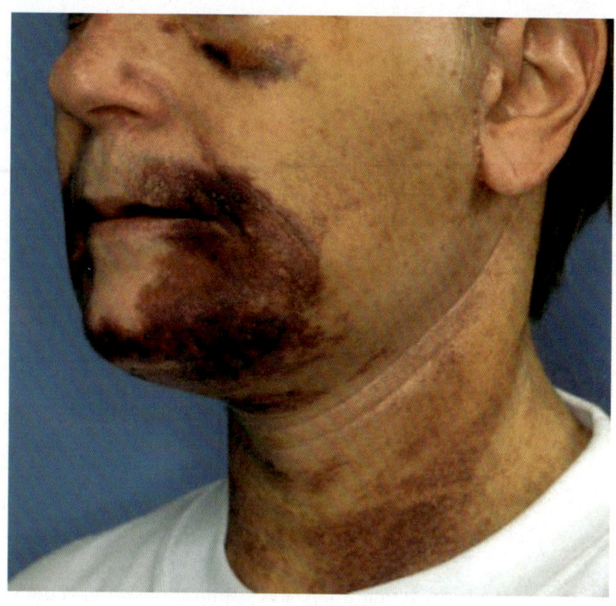

Figure 5-1. Marked ecchymoses in a patient who did not stop daily ASA preoperatively.

In addition to anticoagulants, aspirin, and NSAIDS, the surgeon should not forget to ask the patient about other herbal remedies or vitamins, including vitamin E, that may promote coagulation difficulties.

Infection

Infection is a reported but rare complication in facelift patients. Should it be encountered, most patients will respond rapidly to wound drainage and continued oral antibiotics. Antibiotic therapy should be guided by a culture. Typically infection is heralded by redness, swelling, fluctuation, possible localized pain, and wound drainage. These may be secondary sequelae to unrecognized hematoma or seroma.

Nerve Damage

Patients should be warned that nearly all individuals will experience some hypoesthesia for 4–12 weeks following facelift surgery; this is an expected sequelae rather than a complication. Loss of sensation for longer periods may indicate division or ligation of a portion of the auricular nerve. Although unusual, this nevertheless is reported as the most commonly injured nerve in facelift surgery. It is likely more commonly injured by monopolar cautery than by actual division, but division and even ligation may be possible during SMAS or skin-flap elevation. If division of the nerve is recognized at the time of surgery the proximal and distal ends should be reanastamosed by epineural repair using a fine suture (**Figure 5-2**).

Damage to the branches of the seventh cranial or facial nerve creates motor damage and is a significant injury. The most frequent branches are reportedly the margin mandibular or frontal temporal branches. Injuries to the buccal nerve have been reported but should be even more unusual. To date we have experienced no facial nerve injuries following facelift surgery, and we, felt that the Safety Facelift approach as described in this text contribute to a greater margin of safety for our patients. Typically facial nerve injury is not recognized at the time of surgery, and weakness early on may be related to the local anesthetic infiltration. Of course, if one recognizes that a major branch of the facial nerve has been divided, immediate repair should be attempted. More often this is recognized postoperatively, and an anastamosis of the small distal branches of the facial nerve are not practical. Most facial nerve injuries fortunately resolve with time (**Figure 5-3**).

Poor Scars

Widened, depressed, or even hypertrophic scars are possible after facelift procedures. Again, the techniques described in this text should allow for minimal tension on wound closure and thus a tendency

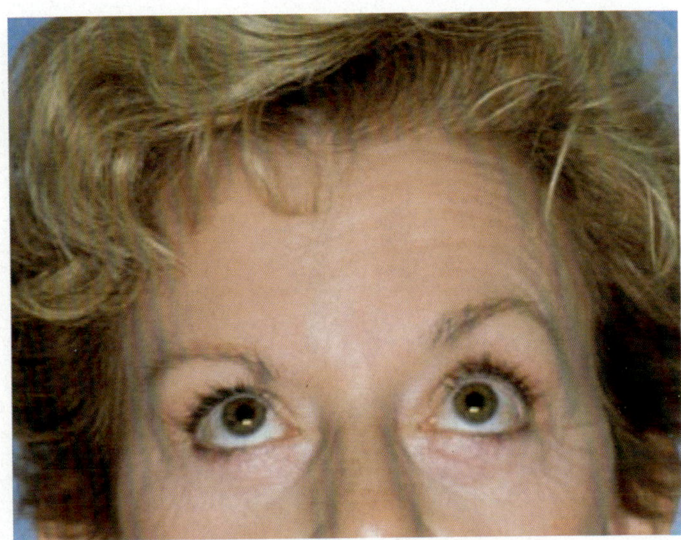

Figure 5-2. A right temporal nerve injury in a patient whose surgeon extended dissection to the orbital rim region.

for better, more acceptable scars. Similarly, appropriate scar placement that hides scars in appropriately camouflage positions should further diminish issues of scar appearance postoperatively (**Figure 5-4**).

Should hypertrophic scarring begin to occur, periodic intralesional injection of steroids should be instituted. Typically, triamcinolone 10 mg/cc at 2- to 4-week intervals will suffice at softening and flattening hypertrophic scars. Excision and reclosure of hypertrophic scarring should be delayed 6–8 for months (**Figure 5-5**).

Earlobe deformity related to scarring or pulling on the earlobe region is often referred to as "satyr's ear" or "pixie ear." This typically is related to poor incision placement or subsequent scarring beneath the earlobe, which can displace the lobe itself. Prevention is the best step to avoid this, of course. The treatment can include resection of the scar near the lobe and advancement beneath the lobe along with creation of a new earlobe sulcus.

Hair Loss

Actual hair loss is often related to damage to the hair follicles from use of an inappropriate plane of dissection. Hair loss may also be related to use of monopolar cautery and damage to hair follicles in the cautery field. It is wise to use a bipolar cautery, which minimizes that electrical field and thus damages hair follicles, throughout the procedure

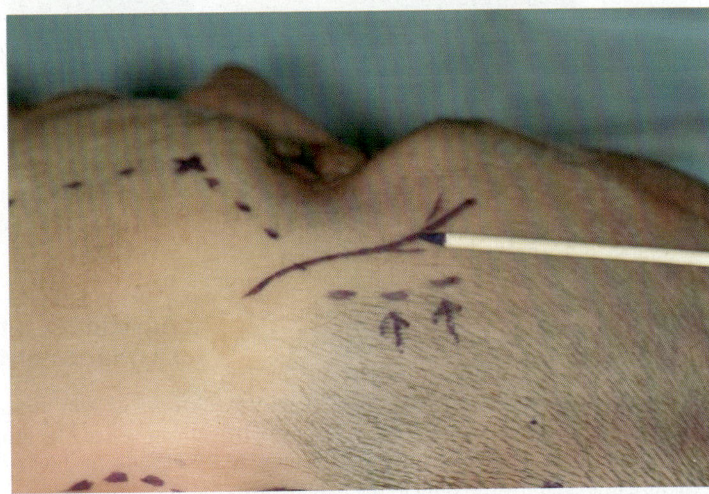

Figure 5-3. Stopping dissection at the temporal hairline avoids the temporal branch of the facial nerve as indicated on the cadaver specimen.

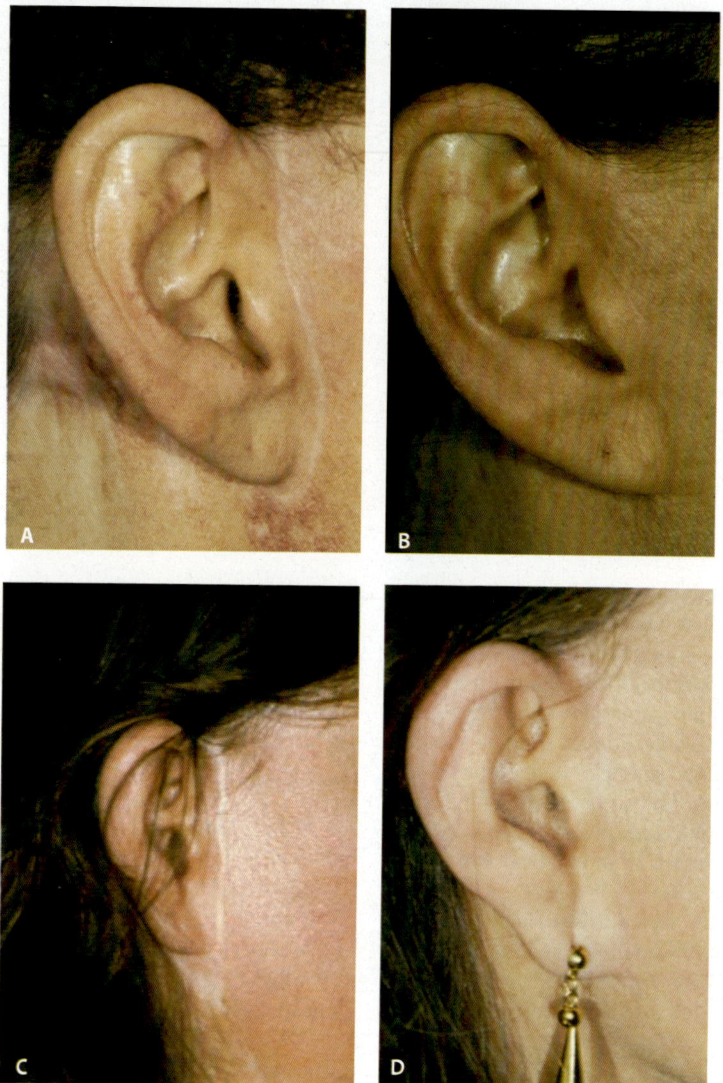

Figure 5-4. A poorly positioned scar (A) is better camouflaged by creating a posttragal advancement (B). Another malpositioned scar (C) is improved by placement in proper area (D).

as well as any other procedures in hair-bearing skin. In areas of hair loss, waiting a period of 3–6 months is appropriate to see if there is a return of hair at that time. It has been suggested that topical minoxidil may be useful in promoting a return of hair. Distortion of the hairline may also be related to inappropriate rotation and advancement of hair-bearing skin, which eliminates the normal hair line and pulls non–hair-bearing skin into its place. This is a problem that can be avoided by using appropriate surgical maneuvers. Failure to recognize this can be distressing to the patient postoperatively and create hairline deformities. Hair transplantation or hair-bearing flap revision may be required postoperatively (**Figures 5-6, 5-7, 5-8, 5-9, 5-10**).

Auricular Cleft and Lobe Displacement

Loss of the infra-auricular cleft below the earlobe can usually be attributed to tension on the wound closure in this region. There should be no tension on skin edges, as the flap is tailored around the

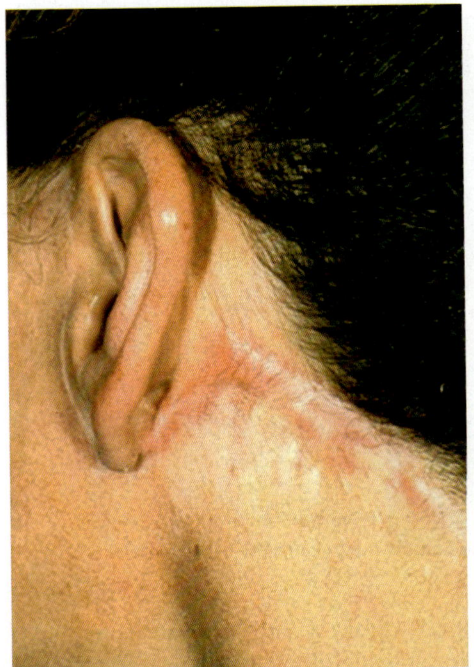

Figure 5-5. A poorly positioned incision with too much tension on the closure creating a hypertrophic scar).

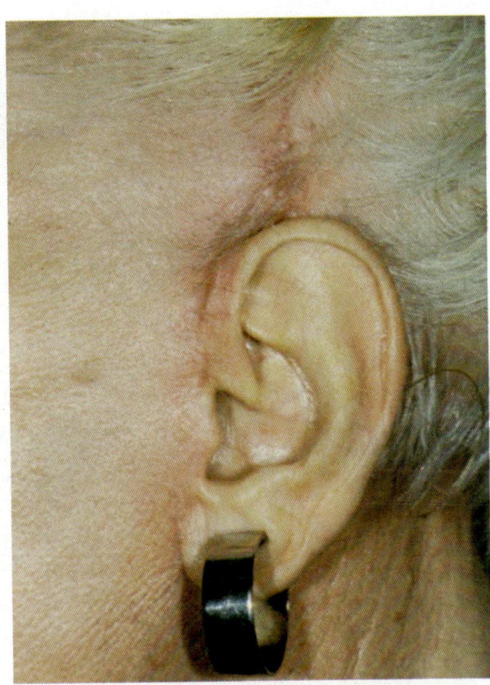

Figure 5-7. Hair loss from a poorly placed incision and too much advancement of temporal skin.

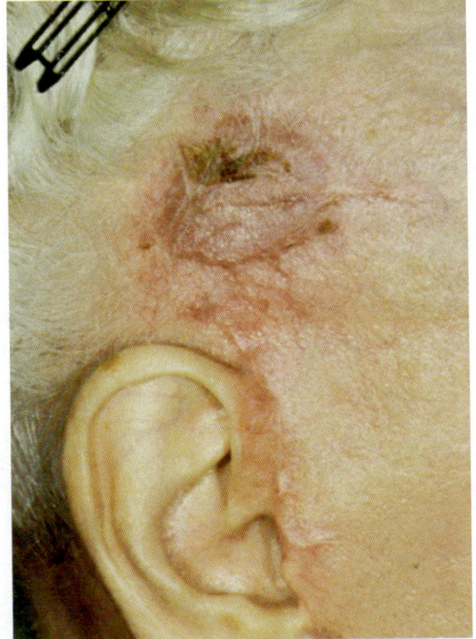

Figure 5-6. Tension on the wound closure creating scarring and hair loss.

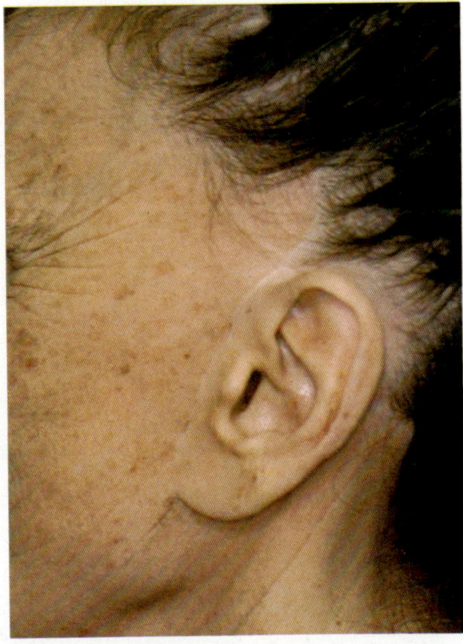

Figure 5-8. Over advancement of skin in a poorly placed temporal incision.

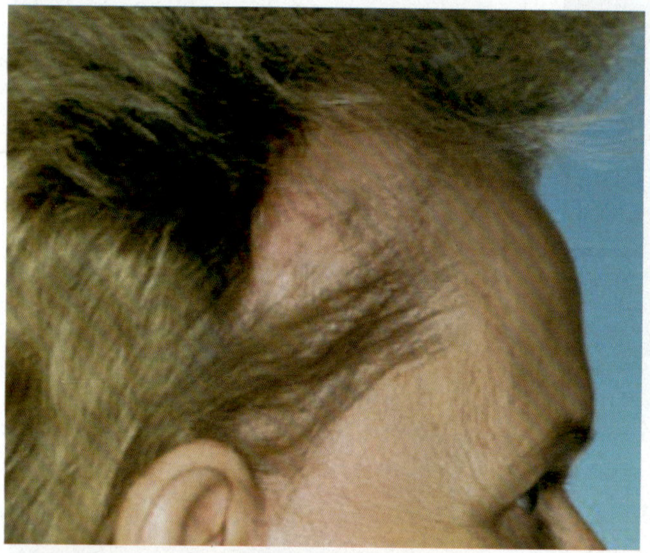

Figure 5-9. Hair loss following surgeon's use of mono polar cautery.

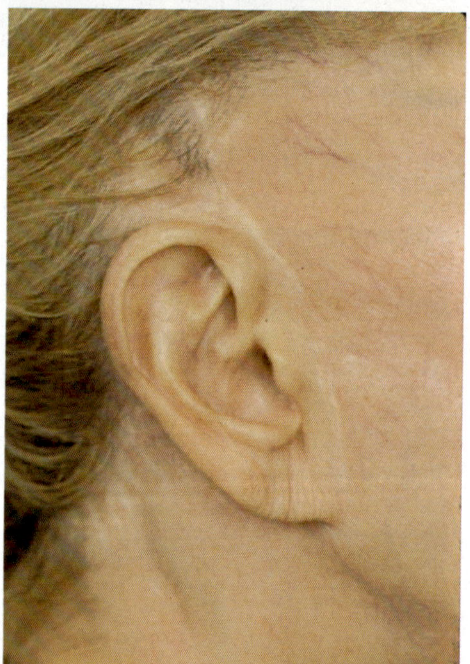

Figure 5-10. Temporal hair loss related to poor incision planning.

auricle. Usually a small amount of bunching of the skin in this region helps ensure that loss of the cleft is avoided. The deformity created by inferiorly directed tension on the earlobe creates a deformity frequently called pixie ear or Satan's ear. Correction entails surgically creating a new cleft dividing the lobe attachment, advancing the cheek skin to a more superior position, and closure. Prevention as always is the preferred axiom.

References

1. Tardy ME, Thomas, JR. *Facial Aesthetic Surgery*. St. Louis, Mosby- Yearbook, 1995.
2. Becker FF, Castellano RD. Safety of face-lifts in the older patient. *Arch Facial Plast Surg*. 2004, 6, 311–314.
3. Jones BM, Grover R. Avoiding hematoma in cervicofacial rhytidectomy: A personal 8 year quest. *Plast Reconstr Surg*. 2004, 113, 381–387.

6

Other Considerations

Ancillary Procedures

It is not unusual to combine other procedures with a facelift, including upper- and lower-lift blepharoplasty, various forms of brow or forehead lifting, and at times rhinoplasty. However, more specific procedures to enhance results of the facelift itself would include chin augmentation and injectable fillers.

Chin Augmentation

A poor jawline is manifested by facial disharmony in proportion and balance.[1,2] An elegant strong jawline is perhaps the most desirable feature in gaining optimum facelift results. Also important are appropriate skin tone and the presence of adipose. Inadequate chin projection may be improved through chin augmentation. The facelift surgeon will find that a stronger chin will enhance the submental appearance and the ability to further improve the jawline. The chin implant can be placed and positioned through the submental incision that is used for platysmal plication and submental liposuction.

A variety of materials are available for chin augmentation.[3] Due to the fixed soft-tissue coverage, good vascularity, and the ability to immobilize the area, the chin is an appropriate area for alloplastic materials. Placement of the implant is accomplished through dissection down to the periosteum overlaying the mandible. Surgical judgment must be used in terms of selecting the size and shape of the implant to be used. A central strip of intact periosteum is left intact to help prevent bony erosion. Two lateral subperiosteal pockets are formed precisely. Once these precise pockets have been developed, the implant is put into place. Typically, one to two absorbable sutures are placed through the implant to the periosteal tissue to further immobilize the implant during healing. The implant is soaked in an antibiotic solution before placement. After placement, the wound is irrigated with an antibiotic irrigation solution and the wound is closed in multiple layers. The chin region is immobilized with tape dressing postoperatively for several days and the incision is incorporated in the facelift dressing.

Injectable Augmentation

Regardless of the technique used, the nasolabial or melolabial fold regions may not be effaced or corrected through the surgical intervention. These areas are often are treated either at the time of surgery or during the perioperative period with one of the many injectable augmentation materials available. Choice of materials is based on the surgeons' preference, the patient's wishes, and the anticipated desire for persistence of the material before the need for reaugmentation. There are numerous approved materials available on the market and selection should be discussed preoperatively with the patient. These injectable materials can greatly enhance the facelift results.

Chin Augmentation as an Adjunct to Rhytidectomy

Background

Augmentation of the chin, or mentoplasty, is useful both as a standalone procedure and as an adjunct that may enhance the results of a rhinoplasty or rhytidectomy. The surgeon should always assess patients undergoing rhytidectomy for chin deficiency. A chin deficiency can be classified as either retrognathia or microgenia depending on the etiology. Retrognathia refers to a small chin due to an underlying skeletal deformity and may be accompanied by abnormal occlusion. Conversely, microgenia describes a small chin in the absence of a skeletal or occlusal deformity. A patient with neck laxity, jowling, and a chin deficiency will benefit from either genioplasty or mentoplasty concurrently with a rhytidectomy to achieve the most aesthetic jawline and cervicomental angle. Additionally, some candidates for rhytidectomy with anteroinferiorly positioned hyoids will also benefit from chin augmentation even in the absence of a true chin deficiency.

Although the terms genioplasty and mentoplasty are sometimes used synonymously, genioplasty more often refers to procedures that involve true osseous advancement. Mentoplasty generally implies the use of an alloplastic implant to increase chin projection.[4] We prefer mentoplasty with a silastic implant to osseous techniques because implants are easier to place, can be carved with greater precision, are associated with fewer complications, and are completely reversible. Our extensive experience with alloplastic augmentation has also biased us toward this approach. Complications of osseous genioplasty can include mental nerve injury, malunion, nonunion, irregularity, step deformities, asymmetry, irreversibility, and lip drop.[4] Risks may be further increased in the setting of decreased mandibular bone mass encountered frequently in the aging female population that typically undergoes rhytidectomy. The majority of patients needing chin augmentation are deficient primarily in the sagittal plane, and alloplastic implants are ideal for this type of deficiency. Other patients may have a weak jawline laterally in the axial plane due to bilateral prejowl deficiencies. Specialized chin implants that primarily enhance the prejowl areas are effective for these patients as well. The occasional patient has concurrent malocclusion or is malproportioned in the coronal plane, described as vertical macro- or microgenia. Dental evaluation and osseous techniques are indicated for vertical disproportion, and alloplastic augmentation is neither beneficial nor appropriate in this population.[5]

Patient Selection

The patient with a deficient chin who undergoes rhytidectomy will not achieve the optimal result unless the surgeon addresses the chin simultaneously. Meticulous preoperative analysis is the key to identifying the subset of rhytidectomy candidates that will benefit from adjunctive mentoplasty.

Several methods are used to evaluate chin aesthetics. Surgeons skilled in orthognathic procedures often prefer cephalometry, or the use of a radiograph, to assess occlusion and make skeletal measurements. While this is indicated for patients needing orthognathic or dental work, obtaining a radiograph for the patient who desires only an aesthetic correction is usually unnecessary. However, even patients who are uninterested in orthognathic surgery deserve a thorough preoperative exam that includes inspection of bite and occlusion. Ideally the mesiobuccal cusp of the first maxillary molar sits in the buccal groove of the mandibular first molar; this is called class I occlusion. The most common type of malocclusion seen in association with the deficient chin is class II. In class II occlusion the mesiobuccal cusp of the maxillary first molar rests mesial, or anterior, to the buccal groove of the mandibular first molar. Class II malocclusion defines true retrognathia. Patients with retrognathia and malocclusion may be unaware of the dental abnormality and should at least be offered a referral for dental evaluation. Patients that have no occlusal abnormalities or that are uninterested in pursuing dental devaluation can be adequately evaluated for mentoplasty in the clinic using soft-tissue landmarks alone.

After occlusal abnormalities have been ruled out or addressed, evaluating the chin's relationship to applicable soft tissue landmarks with an appreciation for aesthetic ideals is essential. Useful anatomic landmarks for assessing sagittal chin deficiency include the nasion, subnasale, stomion, vermillion border of the lower lip, pogonion, and menton. The pogonion is defined as the most anterior point of the chin and should project to a line dropped from the lower lip vermillion border that is perpendicular to the Frankfort horizontal. In women, it is also acceptable for the pogonion to lie up to 2 mm behind this line (**Figure 6-1**).[6] Alternatively, a line can be dropped from the nasion that is perpendicular to the Frankfort horizontal, and again the pogonion should approximate this line.[7] The chin should not only project adequately from a lateral view but also be full enough laterally in the axial plane to define a strong jawline from a frontal view. Prejowl deficiency is diagnosed in the absence of a smooth transition inferiorly from the mentum to the body of the mandible. Aging frequently results in gradual resorption along the inferior border of the mandible in the areas immediately anterior to the jowls, disrupting the jawline.[8] A patient with prejowl deficiency may be a candidate for a specialized chin implant that fills

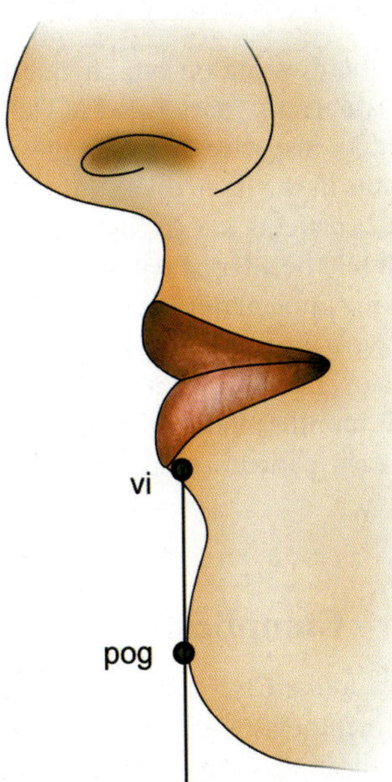

Figure 6-1. A line perpendicular to the Frankfort horizontal is dropped from the vermillion border of the lower lip (VI). The pogonion (Pog) should approximate this line. In women, the pogonion may lie up to 2 mm behind this line.

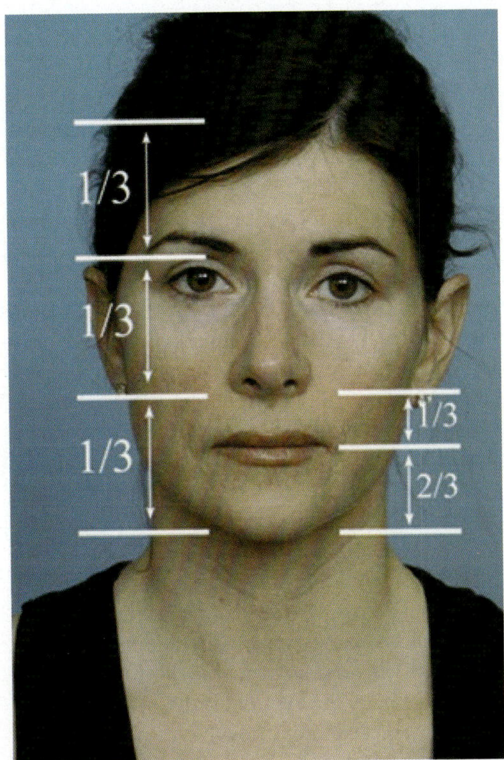

Figure 6-2. When evaluating vertical proportions of the chin, ideally the distance from the level of the menton (Me) to the stomion (St) is twice as great as the distance from the stomion (St) to the subnasale (Sn). In reference to the vertical proportions of the entire face, the total distance from the subnasale to the menton should approximate the distance from the hairline to the nasion (Na) as well as the distance from the nasion to the subnasale.

the prejowl areas with minimal or no augmentation of the mandible in the midline. Finally, the vertical dimension of the chin should be analyzed as well. In the coronal plane on a frontal view, the lower third of the face should be proportioned such that the distance from the level of the menton to the stomion is twice as great as the distance from the stomion to the subnasale **(Figure 6-2)**.[7] A patient found to have a significant vertical deficiency should be offered orthognathic intervention and will not benefit from alloplastic augmentation.

Surgical Technique

Preoperative Preparation

Patients are marked in the preoperative area as needed for rhytidectomy. No additional markings are necessary for concurrent mentoplasty to be performed. The procedure can be performed under general anesthesia or with local infiltration and intravenous sedation. If an endotracheal tube is to be used, it is worthwhile to have a preoperative discussion with the anesthesiologist regarding how the tube will be secured so that it will neither distort nor impede access to the chin. Once the patient is asleep or sedated, we inject 1% lidocaine with 1:100,000 epinephrine at our submental incision site and along the inferior border of the mandible. Inferior alveolar nerve blocks may be useful as well if the procedure is to be done under sedation.

TABLE 6-1 Chin Implant Enhancements
1. Improved chin projection
2. Enhanced cervicomental angle
3. Better repositioning of soft-tissue rectors
4. Balanced facial relationships and proportions

Mentoplasty

Chin augmentation is performed following submental liposuction and platysmal plication but prior to lateral SMAS imbrication when combined with rhytidectomy. If an incision has been made for liposuction or platysmal plication, it can be extended slightly to accommodate a chin implant. Otherwise, a 2- to 3-cm submental incision is made with a #15 blade. Although a transoral gingivolabial sulcus incision can also be used for placement of the chin implant, we believe the risks of implant migration superiorly and salivary leak into the neck outweigh the benefits of this approach. Certainly the submental approach is superior when performing concurrent rhytidectomy, as the same incision can be used for both procedures. After making the incision, dissection is performed sharply down to the mandibular periosteum. The midline of the mandible is identified, and two 10 mm vertical incisions are made through the periosteum at the mandible's inferior border that are 5 mm lateral to the midline on either side, leaving a 10-mm segment of attached periosteum crossing the midline between the two incisions. The periosteum in the midline is left undisturbed, whereas bilateral subperiosteal pockets are developed along the inferior border of the mandible using the Freer elevator through each periosteal incision. These subperiosteal pockets must be symmetrical and just large enough to accommodate the implant in order to prevent later migration. One should be aware of the inferior alveolar nerve, but, even in the aging mandible, the nerve should not be encountered if dissection remains within 8 mm of the inferior mandibular border in the region of the mental foramen.[8] The nerve always exits lateral to the canines and only a small pocket is required in this area to accommodate the laterally tapered implant. For sagittal chin deficiency, we prefer to use an extended anatomic silastic implant because of its natural appearance, nonreactivity, and ease of removal when necessary. Typically either the "small-" or "medium-" sized implant is used. The implant is secured into place in the midline with one or two 4-0 polydioxanone (PDS) sutures placed both through the implant and through the attached midline mandibular periosteum. A few simple buried 5-0 PDS stitches are placed to provide subcutaneous coverage of the implant. Interrupted 6-0 Prolene is then used to close the skin. (**Figure 6-3**) shows step-by-step drawings and photographs of our surgical technique. Bacitracin ointment, a piece of sterile nonadherent gauze, and paper tape are placed over the incision. If you are placing an elastic or pressure dressing after a rhytidectomy, inspect the dressing closely to see that it is not displacing the chin implant.

Postoperative Care

We change the dressing on our rhytidectomy patients on postoperative days 1 and 2. The chin implant should be inspected at these times to ensure that it remains in the desired location. On postoperative day 2, patients are given an elastic facelift strap and should be advised not to allow it to place pressure on the implant during wear. All sutures are removed 1 week postoperatively. We schedule additional postoperative visits at 2 weeks, 1 month, 3 months, 6 months, and 1 year; although, this is tailored to each patient's individual schedule and needs.

Complications

Few complications are typically observed in patients undergoing mentoplasty. Rubin and Yaremchuk reviewed complications of implantable material and found a 1.4% infection rate for chin implants. They also found a 0.5 % rate of displacement.[9] We have encountered a similar infrequent rate of infection, although an implant inevitably must be removed if this occurs. Displacement is rare especially when the implant is inserted into a tight pocket and secured with suture to the mandibular periosteum. Occasional temporary lower-lip numbness occurs presumably due to tension placed on the mental nerves during subperiosteal dissection. Late complications are unusual unless a laceration or other trauma results in implant exposure. Patients should be counseled that there is the potential for bone resorption at the pogonion after many years; however, most patients do not lose soft tissue projection of the chin with even several millimeters of bony resorption.[6]

Summary

In rhytidectomy candidates with chin deficiency, an optimal jawline and cervicomental angle cannot be achieved without addressing this deficiency. We find that mentoplasty with an alloplastic implant is a useful adjunct to rhytidectomy when either a sagittal or prejowl chin deficiency is present. Vertical deficiency is more appropriately addressed with osseous techniques. When indicated, mentoplasty is readily combined with a rhytidectomy through a submental approach, is associated with few complications, and will increase the satisfaction of appropriately selected patients.

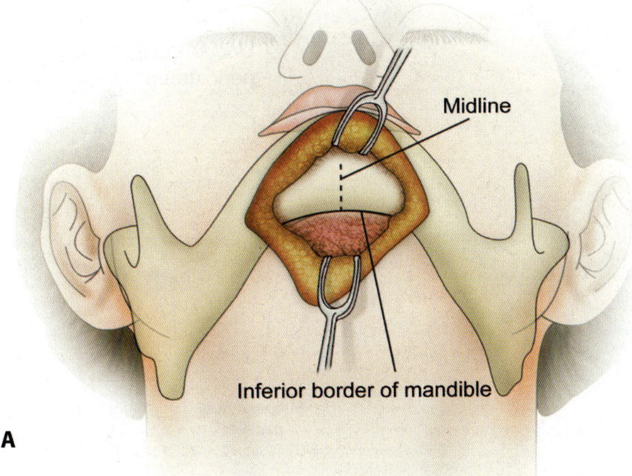

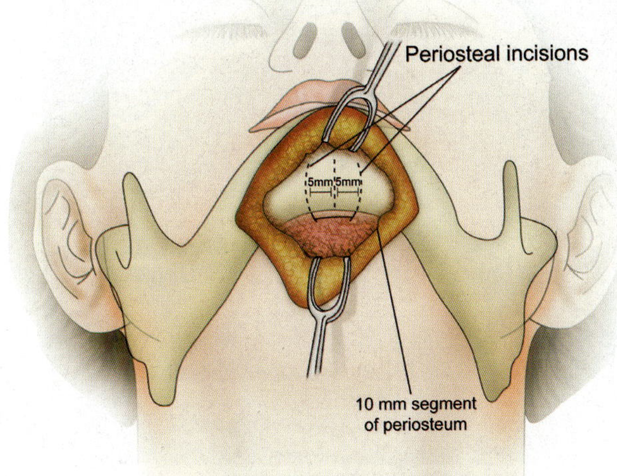

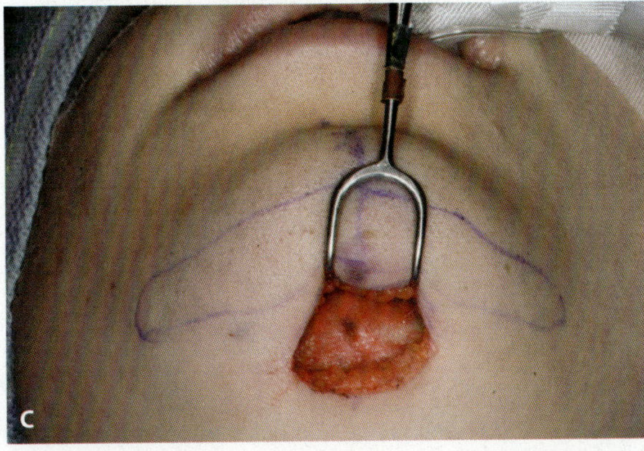

Figure 6-3. After a submental incision centered on the midline is made, subcutaneous dissection is performed down to the mandibular periosteum. The midline and the inferior border of the mandible are identified. Bilateral vertical periosteal incisions are made 5 mm from the midline and 1 cm long (A,B,C). *(Continued)*

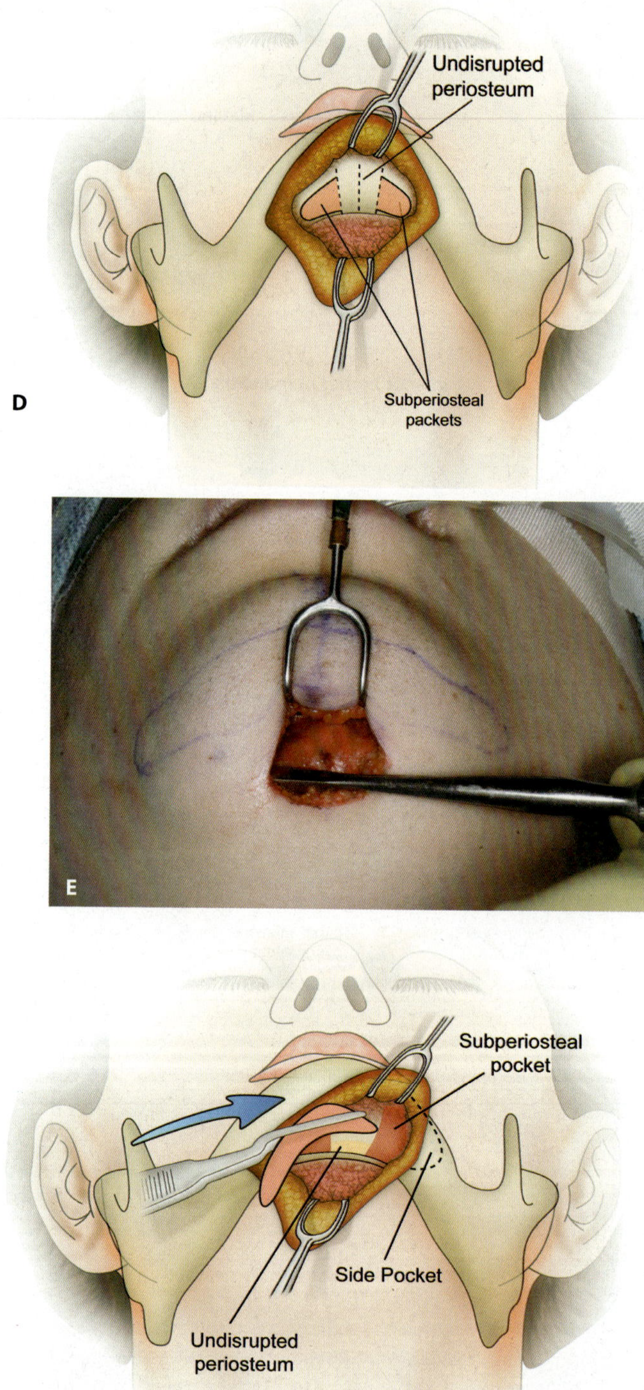

Figure 6-3. *(Continued)* Periosteal pockets are developed along the inferior border of the mandible to accommodate the implant (D,E) Both ends of the implant are inserted into the pockets. The fit should be snug to prevent migration (F,G,H).

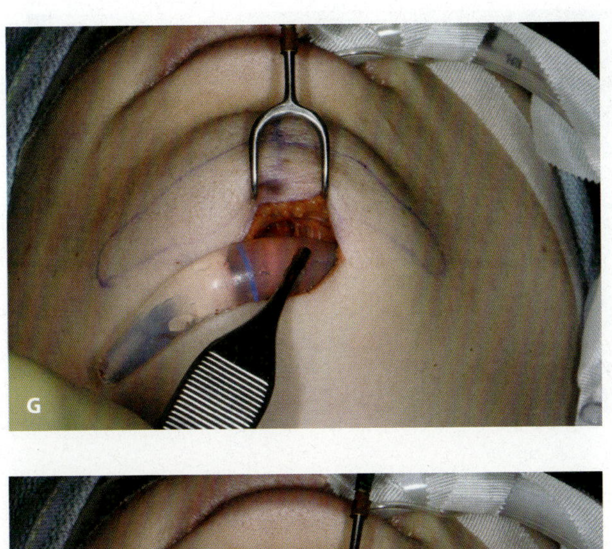

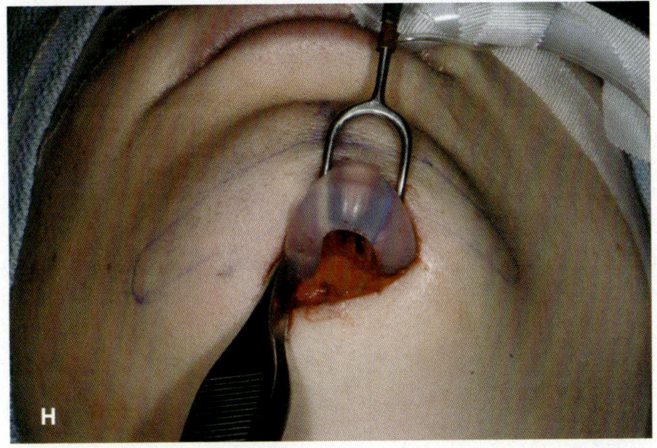

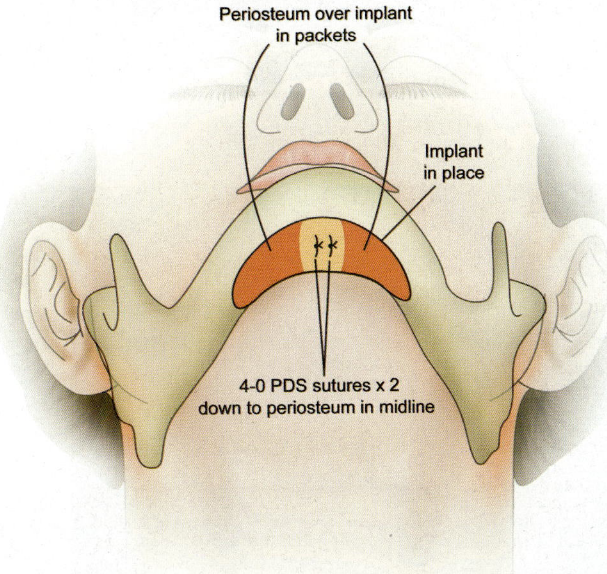

Figure 6-3. *(Continued)* One or two 4-0 PDS sutures are placed to anchor the implant to the mandibular periosteum near the midline (I,J).

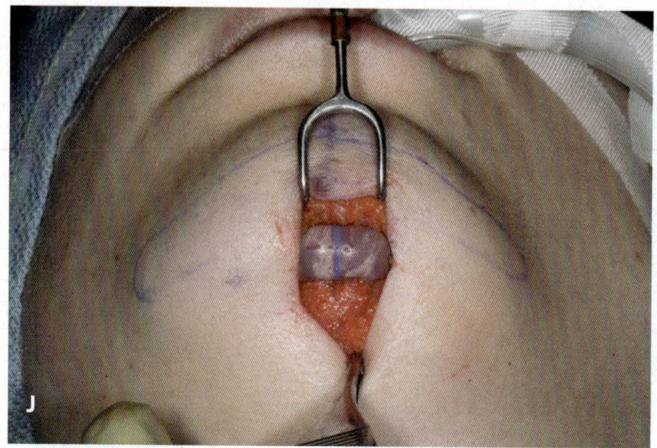

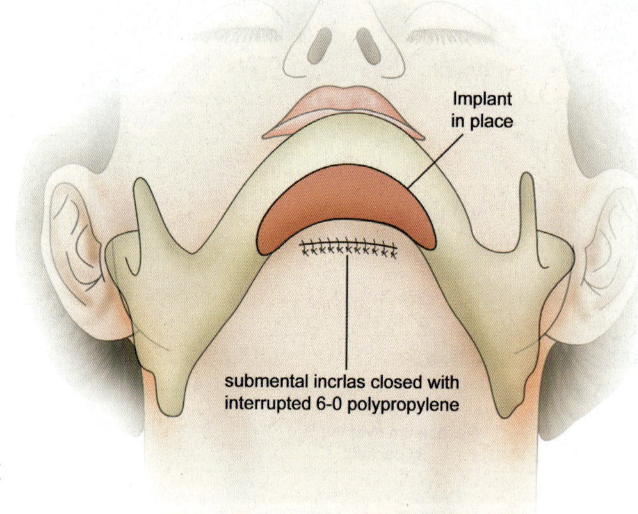

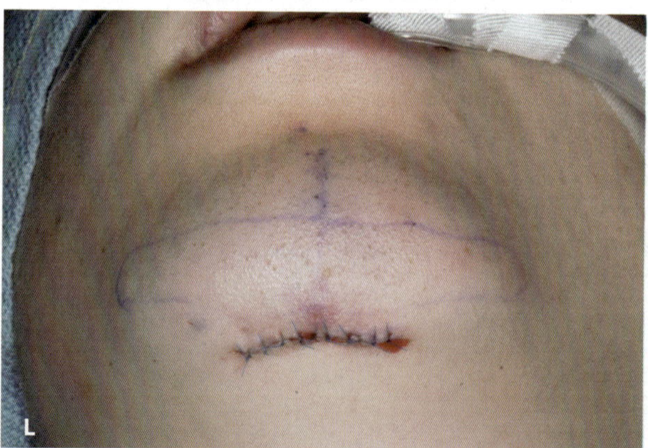

Figure 6-3. *(Continued)* Layered closure is performed using a 5-0 PDS to reapproximate the fascia and subcutaneous tissue followed by interrupted 6-0 Prolene to reapproximate the skin (K,L).

References

1. Powell N, Humphreys B. *Proportions of the Aesthetic Face*. New York, Thieme Stratton, 1984.
2. Thomas JR. Analysis of patient response to preoperative computerized video imaging. *Arch Otol Head Neck Surg*. 1989, 115, 793–796.
3. Mittelman H, Newman J. Aesthetic mandibular implants. In ID Papel, ed., *Facial Plastic and Reconstructive Surgery*. New York, Thieme 2002.
4. Chang EW, Lam SM, Karen M, Donlevy JL. Sliding genioplasty for correction of chin abnormalities. *Arch Facial Plast Surg*. 2001;3:8–15.
5. Frodel JL, Sykes JM, Jones JL. Evaluation and treatment of vertical microgenia. *Arch Facial Plast Surg*. 2004, 6, 111–119.
6. Romo T, Lanson BG. Chin augmentation. *Facial Plast Surg Clin N Am*. 2008, 16, 69–77.
7. Perkins SW, Sandel HD. Anatomic considerations, analysis, and the aging process of the perioral region. *Facial Plast Surg Clin N Am*. 2007, 15, 403–407.
8. Mittelman H, Spencer JR, Chrzanowski DS. Chin region: Management of grooves and mandibular hypoplasia. *Facial Plast Surg Clin N Am*. 2007, 15, 445–460.
9. Rubin JP, Yaremchuk MJ. Complications and toxicities of implantable biomaterials used in facial reconstructive and aesthetic surgery: A comprehensive review of the literature. *Plast Recontr Surg*. 1997, 100, 1336–1353.

7

Small-Incision Rhytidectomy

Background

The demand for facial aesthetic surgery has surged over the past two decades. This increased demand is, in part, due to interest in surgical rejuvenation within a younger population.[1] Less aggressive rhytidectomy techniques can be effective in this typically active population whose goals are minimal risk, rapid recovery, and meaningful results. Small-incision, or short-scar, rhytidectomy is an alternative to more traditional superficial musculoaponeurotic system (SMAS) and deep-plane techniques for properly selected candidates who desire to minimize downtime while still achieving significant rejuvenation in the face and neck. We have also found the small-incision technique useful as a secondary procedure to maintain correction following a prior traditional rhytidectomy.

A small-incision technique was originally described as early as 1919 by the Parisian surgeon Raymond Passot in his publication *Le chirurgie esthetique des rides du visage* [Cosmetic Surgery for Facial Rhytids]. His technique as illustrated in **Figure 7-1** was also among the earliest descriptions of any type of rhytidectomy. The temporal, preauricular, and postauricular incisions used by Passot are not dissimilar to those still in use today though his suspension depended almost exclusively on exci-

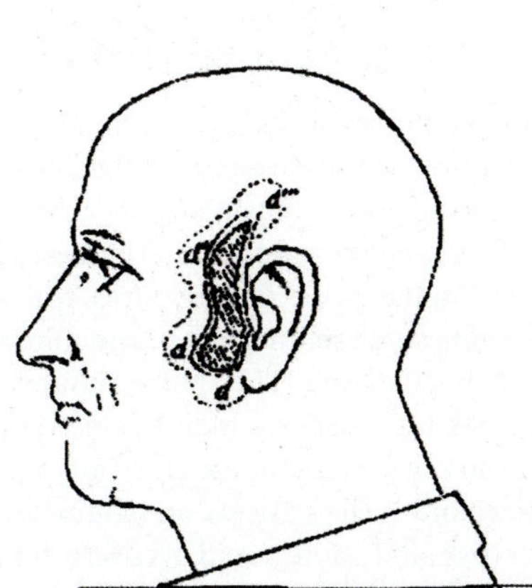
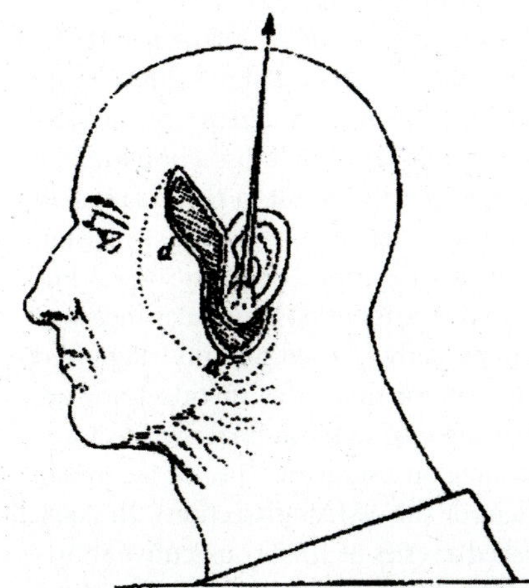

Figure 7-1. Parisian surgeon Raymond Passot published this illustration of his "surgery for facial rhytids" circa 1917. (Reprinted with permission from Brandy DA. A method of augmenting the cheek area through SMAS, sub-SMAS, and subcutaneous tissue recruitment during facelift surgery. *Dermatol Surg.* 2003, 29, 265–271.)

sion and redraping of skin.[2] Improvements on this technique came slowly until advances in anesthesia and an anatomical description of the SMAS by Mitz and Peyronie in 1976 allowed surgeons to safely perform more extensive dissections and relieve tension placed on the skin.[3] SMAS plication, or imbrication with or without sub-SMAS dissection anterior to the parotid gland, soon became the gold standard for rhytidectomy. In 1990, Hamra described the deep-plane technique that carried dissection further medially over the zygomaticus muscles in an attempt to mobilize the malar fat pad.[4] Advocates of these progressively more aggressive techniques claim enhanced midface improvement but greater intraoperative risk to facial nerve branches, and persistent postoperative edema that prolongs recovery are significant potential disadvantages. Furthermore, recent studies have shown that SMAS plication alone may provide equivalent improvement in the melolabial fold, jowl, and cheek areas when compared with deep-plane rhytidectomy for patients less than 70 years of age.[5]

In stark contrast to the 1980s and 1990s, a trend has emerged over the past 10 years with many surgeons describing their techniques for performing limited rhytidectomies and abandoning more aggressive techniques. Salyan described his "S-lift" in 1999, touting several advantages including short operative time, a rapid recovery period, minimal scarring, low risk, and more natural results. The S-lift consisted of a dual-suture SMAS plication performed through a preauricular incision.[6] Massiha described a SMAS imbrication lift through a preauricular J-shaped incision. He advocates limited subcutaneous dissection to maintain attachments between the SMAS and skin with a more extensive sub-SMAS dissection anterior to the sternocleidomastoid. Massiha avoids dissection into the posterior triangle that will result in redundant skin that necessitates an extended postauricular incision for excision.[7] Baker describes a similar SMAS imbrication technique without postauricular incisions that he uses in properly selected patients.[8] Reported complication rates for short-scar rhytidectomy are comparable or superior to traditional rhytidectomy and are dependent on a surgeon's specific technique (e.g., the extent of sub-SMAS dissection). In 2008, Tanna published a series of 1000 consecutive short-scar rhytidectomies with SMAS plication through a limited pre- and postauricular incision combined with cervicofacial liposuction. Hematoma was the most common major complication in this series, occurring in 1% of patients, and there were no cases of facial nerve injury.[9]

The development, popularity, and effectiveness of legitimate small-incision techniques have also spurred the development of several branded and heavily marketed skin and thread lifts that promise similar results. Little research or evidence exists to demonstrate whether these techniques do or do not work. However, the collective experience over the past 30 years would seem to suggest that any lift that does not rely firmly on principles of SMAS dissection and translocation is unlikely to provide a long-lasting result.

After using various methods including the deep-plane technique over the past two decades, we have found that SMAS imbrication provides the maximum risk to benefit ratio for our patients. Our standard rhytidectomy involves submental liposuction; platysmal plication; temporal, posttragal, and postauricular incisions, and SMAS imbrication along two vectors up to the zygomatic arch and back to the thick postauricular fascia. This is easily modified to a small-incision technique with more limited subcutaneous undermining and SMAS imbrication focused on improvement in the jowls and jawline. An incision that extends from a preauricular point just inferior to the tragus, hugs the conchal cartilage under the lobule, continues postauricular just anterior to the sulcus, and extends to the hairline at the level of the external auditory canal is used (**Figure 7-2**). To avoid a preauricular incision, extending an incision into or along the hairline, and dissecting over the zygoma and anterior to the parotid is feasible for properly selected patients.

Patient Selection

Although the small-incision technique will yield some degree of improvement in the jowls and jawline for a wide range of patients, we achieve our best results in a select population. The best candidates are aged in the forties or early fifties with mild jowl formation, some submental fat, and minimal banding of the platysma. The small-incision technique also lends itself well to candidates needing secondary or so called "tuck-up" surgery following a prior rhytidectomy. The patients are counseled that the lower risk and more rapid recovery time for the procedure are tradeoffs for a result that may last 4–6 years at best. We expect a visible result to persist up to 8 years for our traditional rhytidectomy with a more extensive skin and SMAS dissection. Patients

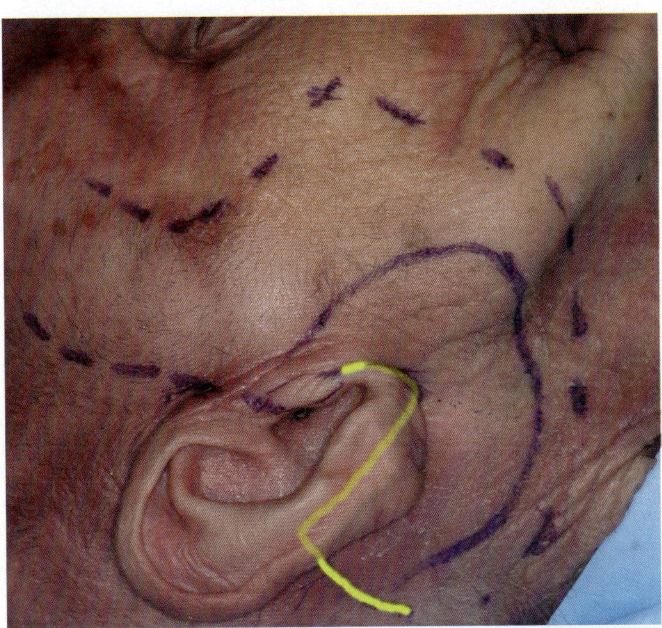

Figure 7-2. A yellow mark demonstrates incision placement just inferior to the tragus, under the lobule, and extending anterior to the postauricular sulcus along the conchal cartilage. The incision is extended to the hairline behind the auricle at the level of the external auditory canal. Translucent portions of the yellow mark indicate incision segments that are hidden by the ear.

who are smokers, diabetics, or have other medical problems are counseled about additional risks, but, in general, the less invasive short-scar technique leads to fewer healing problems due to the reduced dissection and shorter skin flap.

Surgical Technique

Patients are marked in the preoperative area with incision sites and areas to be undermined. Hair is placed in rubber bands to provide adequate exposure for the short-scar technique. The procedure can be performed under general anesthesia or with local infiltration and intravenous sedation. We use 1% lidocaine and 1:100,000 epinephrine for injection along the periauricular and submental incision lines.

After vasoconstriction occurs, submental liposuction is performed first if required. We incise 5–6 mm in the central portion of the submental region with a #15 blade. The incision is just large enough to allow easy passage of the liposuction cannula without traumatizing the skin while maintaining negative pressure. Radiating fanlike tunnels are made over the platysma and extended into the jowls with a 2-mm round cannula without suction applied. A 3-mm beveled spatula cannula is then inserted with the slot facing away from the skin, and suction is activated once the cannula tip is through the incision (**Figure 7-3**). The right hand moves the cannula back and forth while the fingertips of the left hand are used to palpate and direct fat into the tip. The slot, or cannula opening, should always face away from the skin, as suctioning directly on the dermis increases the potential for uneven healing. Once an adequate suction lipectomy has been performed, the remainder of the submental incision is opened with a #15 blade if platysmal banding is present. Usually, a 2.5- to 3-cm incision is adequate to visualize and address the platysma. The medial edges of the platysma are visualized and undermined, developing platysmal flaps. The platysma is then sutured together in the midline with 5-0 polydioxanone suture in a simple running fashion. The submental incision is closed with interrupted 6-0 polypropylene.

After submental liposuction and platysma plication, attention is turned to the periauricular incision. The incision extends from just inferior to the tragus, immediately adjacent to the conchal cartilage under the lobule, anterior to the postauricular sulcus, and back to the hairline at the level of the external auditory canal (**Figure 7-2**). Kaye scissors and Freeman rhytidectomy scissors are used to undermine in a subcutaneous plane 3–4 cm anteriorly and inferiorly from the incision (**Figure 7-4**). A short SMAS flap is also developed with the scissor dissection for 3–4 cm or just beyond the extent of the subcutaneous undermining (**Figure 7-5**). An Alice clamp is placed on the free proximal edge of the SMAS flap and desired tension is applied to affect change in the jowls

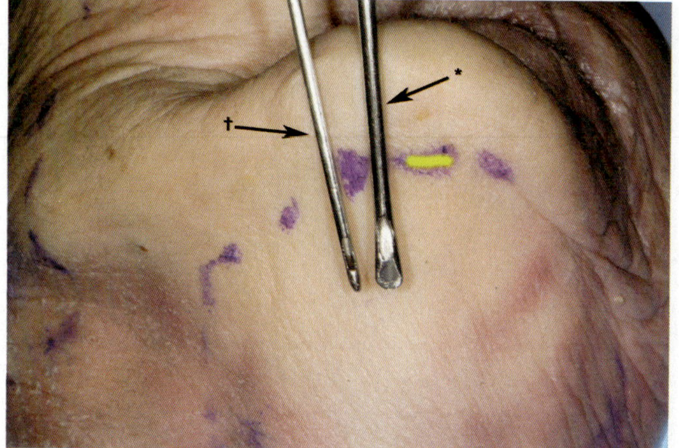

Figure 7-3. A yellow mark demonstrates submental incision placement. An initial 5–6 mm incision will accommodate both the 2- and 3-mm cannulas. The 2-mm round cannula (() is used first to create radiating, fanlike tunnels over the platysma and extended into the jowls without suction. Suction is then applied after inserting a 3-mm beveled spatula cannula (*) with the slot, or opening, facing away from the skin to avoid dermal trauma.

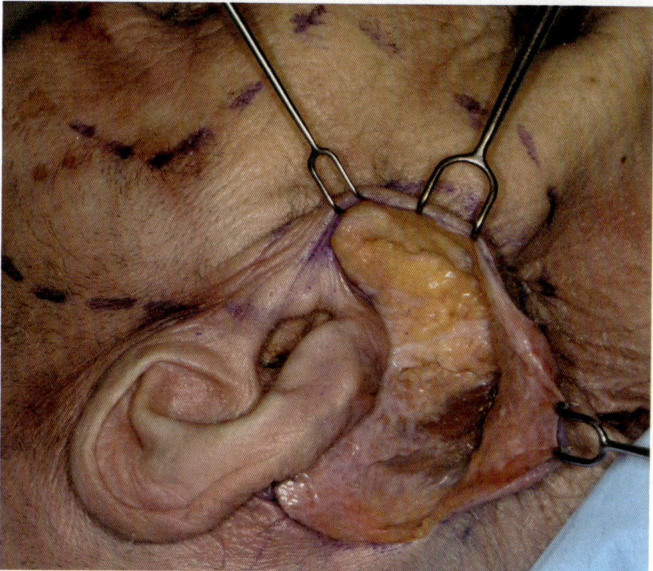

Figure 7-4. Subcutaneous scissor dissection is used to develop a 3- to 4-cm skin flap. The SMAS is visualized lying over the parotid and sternocleidomastoid.

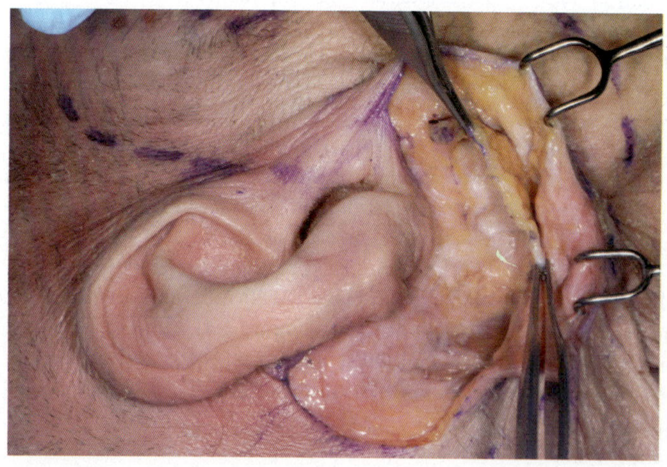

Figure 7-5. The SMAS has been incised and undermined, developing a short flap that can affect change in the jowls and jawline.

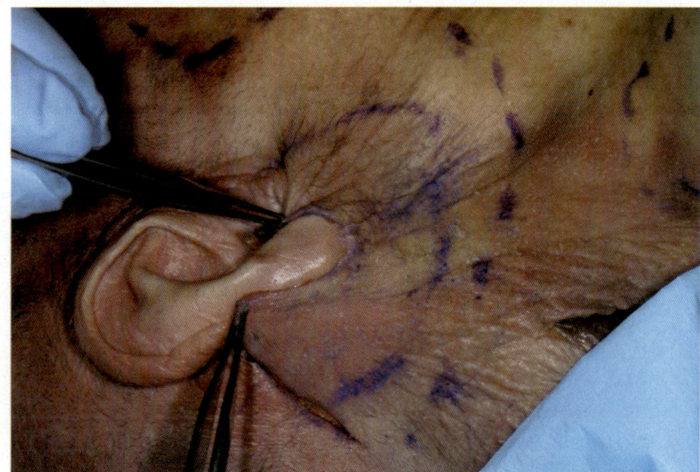

Figure 7-6. After imbrication of the SMAS, the redundant skin flap is redraped.

and jawline. The redundant SMAS is marked and excised. Meticulous hemostasis is achieved using bipolar cauterization. The SMAS is reapproximated and imbrication is completed with interrupted 3-0 polydioxanone. Skin is redraped with minimal tension (**Figure 7-6**) and the excess is trimmed (**Figure 7-7**). We find the postauricular extension of the incision to be essential for adequate skin excision and redraping. Prior to performing skin closure, the proposed opposite side incisions are reinjected using the local anesthetic with a vasoconstrictor. A running, intermittently locked 5-0 fast absorbing gut suture is then used to close the skin incision. The procedure is repeated on the opposite side. At the completion of the procedure, bacitracin ointment is placed liberally over all incision sites. Any rubber bands are removed from the hair. Fluffed gauze is placed over both ears and in the submental area. Four-inch-wide gauze is wrapped from the chin to the vertex and from the forehead to the occiput to secure the dressing. An elastic dressing is then wrapped over the gauze to maintain a moderate degree of pressure. **Figure 7-8** outlines the major steps in the small-incision technique.

Postoperative Care

As with our traditional rhytidectomy patients, we require the patient to be seen on postoperative day 1 to be checked for hematoma and for replacement of the dressing. On postoperative day 2, the dressing is replaced with an elastic facelift strap that the patient can manipulate and change as needed at home. We ask the patient to wear this elastic dressing at all

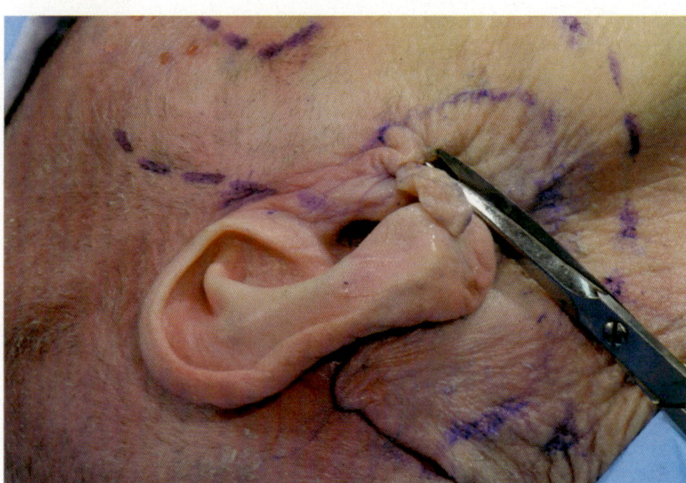

Figure 7-7. Redundant skin is excised with scissors after redraping.

Small-Incision-Stepwise Techniques

1. Local anesthetic/vasoconstrictor infiltration
2. Submental liposuction (A)
3. Platysmal plication (B)
4. Infra- and postauricual incisions (C)
5. Subcutaneous flaps developed (D)
6. SMAS imbrication (E,F)
7. Skin excision and closure (G)
8. Pressure dressing

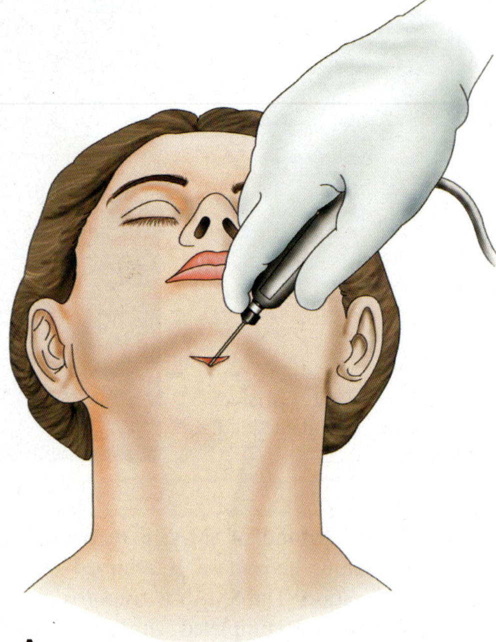

A

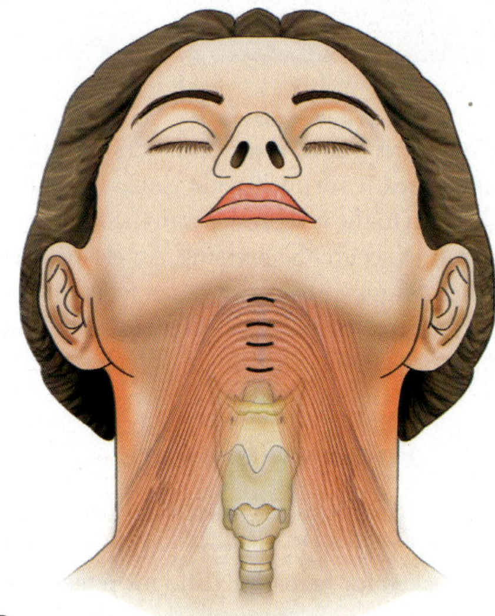

B

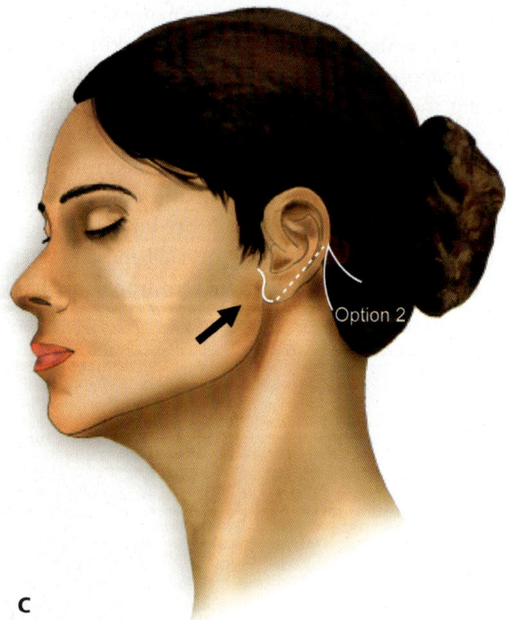

C

Figure 7-8. Major steps in small-incision technique. *(Continued)*

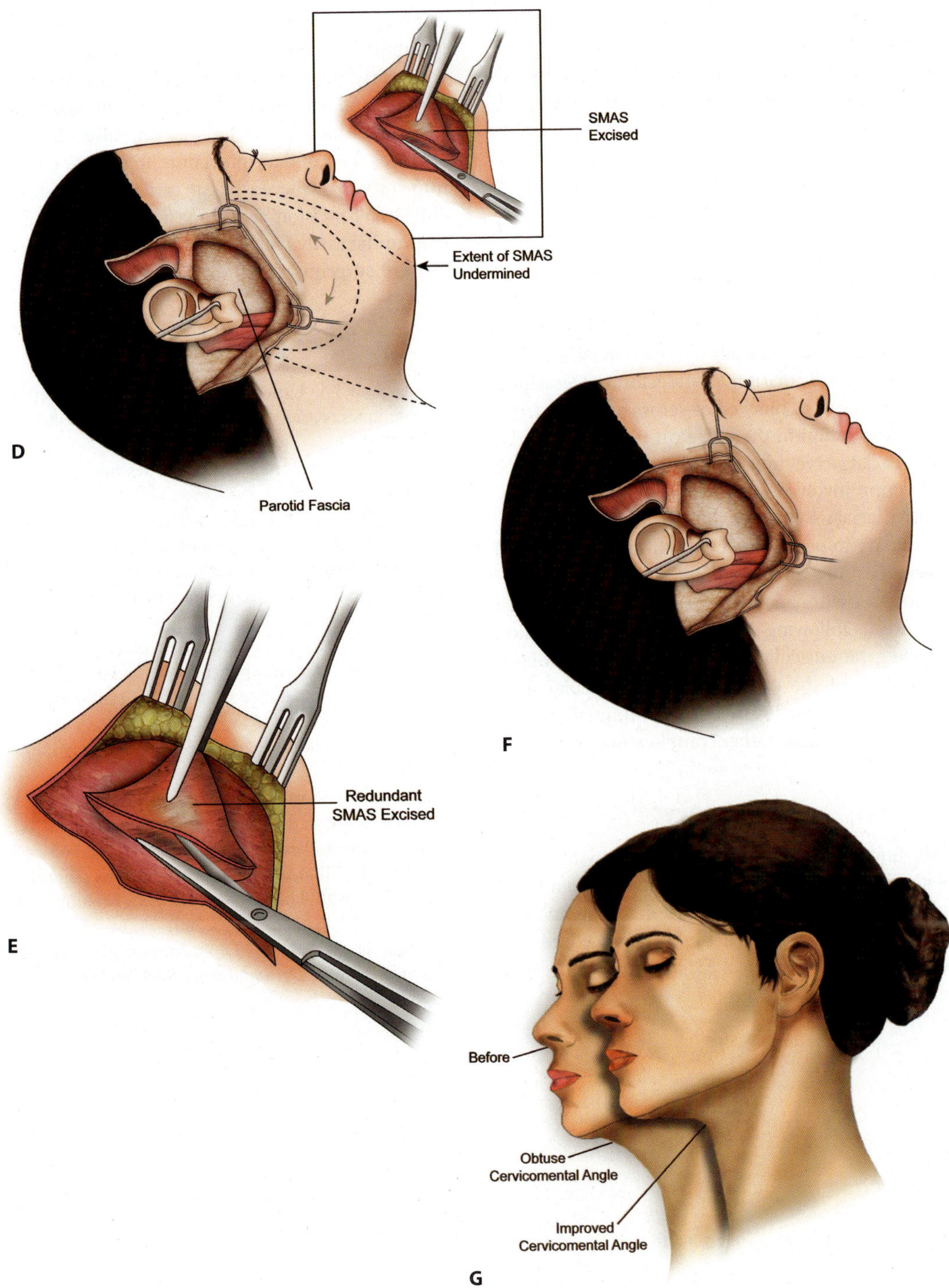

Figure 7-8 *(Continued)*

times if possible for at least 5 days to provide support and promote adherence of the skin flap. The patient wears the elastic dressing at night for an additional week. All sutures are removed 1 week postoperatively. We schedule additional postoperative visits at 2 weeks, 1 month, 3 months, 6 months, and 1 year; although, this is tailored to each patient's individual schedule and needs.

Complications

As with our traditional rhytidectomy technique, few complications are typically observed in patients undergoing small-incision rhytidectomy. Occasional accumulations of blocked or serom are easily treated by aspiration in the office on postoperative day one. Facial nerve injury is unlikely with the limited dissection involved in this procedure, and postoperative facial weakness in the recovery area is usually secondary to persistent activity from the infiltrated lidocaine. All patients should expect to have decreased sensation in the undermined area for at least 6–8 weeks following surgery. Injury or transection of the great auricular nerve can lead to prolonged numbness of the earlobe and postauricular area. Tension-free skin closure ensures minimal scarring along incision sites. Other complications are rare.

Summary

We find that the small-incision rhytidectomy with SMAS plication is a useful adjunct to a facial plastic surgeon's armamentarium. Patients with active lifestyles are amenable to a procedure that offers significant surgical facial rejuvenation with minimal risk and recovery time. The small-incision technique is especially useful in younger patients with early development of jowls, some submental fat, and minimal banding of the platysma. The small-incision technique can also be beneficial as a secondary procedure to restore correction initially achieved by an earlier rhytidectomy. Our small-incision technique is relatively simple and can be easily mastered with rare complications by most surgeons.

References

1. Adamson PA, Litner JA. Evolution of rhytidectomy techniques. *Facial Plast Surg Clin N Am.* 2005, 13, 383–391.
2. Passot R. La chirurigie esthetique des rides du visage. *Presse Med.* 1919, 27, 258–262.
3. MitzV,PeyronieM.Thesuperficialmusculoaponeurotic system (SMAS) in the parotid and cheek area. *Plast Reconstr Surg.* 1976. 58. 80.
4. Hamra ST. The deep-plane rhytidectomy. *Plast Reconstr Surg.*1990, 86, 53–61.
5. Becker FF, Bassichis BA. Deep-plane face-lift vs superficial musculoaponeurotic system plication face-lift: A comparative study. *Arch Facial Plast Surg.* 2004, 6, 8–13.
6. Salyan Z. The S-lift: Less is more. *Aesthetic Surg J.* 1999, 19, 406–409.
7. Massiha H. Short-scar face lift with extended SMAS platysma dissection and lifting and limited skin undermining. *Plast Reconstr Surg* 2003, 112, 663–669.
8. Baker DC. Minimal incision rhytidectomy (short scar face lift) with lateral SMASectomy: Evolution and application. *Aesthetic Surg J.* 2001, 21, 14–26.
9. Tanna N. Review of 1,000 consecutive short-scar rhytidectomies. *Dermatol Surg.* 2008, 34, 196–203.

INDEX

Information in figures and tables is indicated by *f* and *t*.